Urologic Robotic Surgery
in Clinical Practice

T0100579

Prokar Dasgupta
Editor

Urologic Robotic Surgery in Clinical Practice

Foreword by James O. Peabody
and Mani Menon

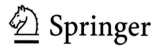 Springer

Editor
Prokar Dasgupta
Department of Urology
Guy's Hospital
London
UK
prokarurol@gmail.com

ISBN: 978-1-84800-242-5   e-ISBN: 978-1-84800-243-2
DOI: 10.1007/978-1-84800-243-2

British Library Cataloguing in Publication Data
A catalogue record for this book is available from the British Library

Library of Congress Control Number: 2008936130

© Springer-Verlag London Limited 2008
Apart from any fair dealing for the purposes of research or private study, or criticism or review, as permitted under the Copyright, Designs and Patents Act 1988, this publication may only be reproduced, stored or transmitted, in any form or by any means, with the prior permission in writing of the publishers, or in the case of reprographic reproduction in accordance with the terms of licenses issued by the Copyright Licensing Agency. Enquiries concerning reproduction outside those terms should be sent to the publishers. The use of registered names, trademarks, etc., in this publication does not imply, even in the absence of a specific statement, that such names are exempt from the relevant laws and regulations and therefore free for general use.
The publisher makes no representation, express or implied, with regard to the accuracy of the information contained in this book and cannot accept any legal responsibility or liability for any errors or omissions that may be made.
Product liability: The publisher can give no guarantee for information about drug dosage and application thereof contained in this book. In every individual case the respective user must check its accuracy by consulting other pharmaceutical literature.

Printed on acid-free paper

Springer Science+Business Media
springer.com

To family, friends, and the science of robotics

Foreword

Computer-enhanced (robotic) surgery is an accepted part of the treatment of various surgical diseases. Since its inception at the turn of this century—8 years ago—robotic-assisted laparoscopic prostatectomy has become the predominant form of surgical treatment for clinically localized prostate cancer in the United States. While robotic-assisted prostatectomy is the first procedure to be performed in great numbers, it is projected that other procedures such as laparoscopic hysterectomy will begin to be performed more commonly with robotic assistance. In fact, most surgical disciplines are beginning to adopt robotic assistance for some of their procedures. Advanced removal and reconstructive procedures are regularly performed in general surgery, head and neck surgery, gynecologic surgery, pediatric surgery, and cardiovascular surgery. The robotic platform that is commonly used (da Vinci™ from Intuitive Surgical) has evolved over the past decade with development of the 4th arm, the tile pro feature, smaller instrumentation and newer instrumentation for specific procedures. It is anticipated that further developments will make this platform and future platforms even easier and more effective to use. Cost remains an extremely important issue for practitioners, hospitals, health plans, and governments as they consider adoption of computer-assisted surgery. This continues to be a barrier to wider adoption of the technology. It is hoped that costs for this equipment will decline as the technology develops and new manufacturers begin to produce robotic platforms, but so far this has not happened.

Professor Dasgupta was among the first in the UK to embrace the use of computer-enhanced (robotic) surgery and his textbook is a timely addition to the field of robotic-assisted urologic surgery. This field has rapidly passed through a period of procedure development and the techniques (with variations) that are presented within the book are now well developed. The chapters cover the most-common procedures in urology that are being performed with contributions by a variety of international experts. In addition, it addresses the important issues of economics and the basic science and technology of robotics.

Surgery is evolving toward less invasive approaches to most procedures and what we have learned through the development of laparoscopic approaches and now computer enhancement should allow for even more minimal access. Multiple instruments will be placed through a single access site and natural orifices will be used as ports of entry. Simulation will allow surgeons to practice the operation before doing it on the patient. Each of these should allow us to do less harm to our patients while we are trying to help them. These are exciting times to be a surgeon.

James O. Peabody MD FACS
and Mani Menon MD FACS
Vattikuti Urology Institute
Henry Ford Health System
Detroit, MI USA

Contents

Contributors

Christopher Anderson
Department of Urology, St Georges Hospital, London, UK
e-mail: cja@blueyonder.co.uk

David Armstrong
Department of General Practice, Kings College London
School of Medicine, London, UK
e-mail: david.armstrong@kcl.ac.uk

Manit Arya
University College Hospital, London, UK
e-mail: manit_arya@yahoo.co.uk

Lisa Blake
Department of Anesthetics, Guy's & St Thomas' NHS
Foundation Trust, London, UK
e-mail: lblake@doctors.org.uk

Ben Challacombe
Department of Urology, Guy's Hospital, London, UK
e-mail: benchallacombe@doctors.net.uk

Mario F. Chammas Jr
Department of Urology, Nancy School of Medicine, Nancy,
France

Anthony J. Costello
Department of Urology, Royal Melbourne Hospital,
Victoria, Australia
e-mail: cosurol@bigpond.net.au

Geoff Coughlin
Center for Robotic & Computer-Assisted Surgery,
Columbus, OH, USA

P. Dasgupta
Department of Urology, Guy's & St Thomas' Hospitals and
King's College London School of Medicine, London, UK
e-mail: prokarurol@gmail.com

Oussama Elhage
Department of Urology, Guy's Hospital, London, UK
e-mail: oelhage@yahoo.com

Sanjay Gulati
Department of Anesthetics, Guy's & St Thomas' NHS
Foundation Trust, London, UK
e-mail: Sanjay.Gulati@gstt.nhs.uk

Nicholas Hegarty
Department of Urology, Guy's Hospital & King's College
London, School of Medicine, London, UK
e-mail: Nicholas.hegarty@hotmail.com

A.K. Hemal
All India Institute of Medical Sciences, New Delhi, India
e-mail: ashokhemal@gmail.com

Panagiotis Kallidonis
Department of Urology, University of Patras, Patras, Greece

Jamie Kearsley
Department of Urology, Royal Melbourne Hospital,
Victoria, Australia
e-mail: jkearsley@urology.org.au

Mohammad Shamim Khan
Department of Urology, Guy's Hospital, London, UK
e-mail: Shamim.khan@gstt.nhs.uk

Roger Kirby
The Prostate Center, London, UK
e-mail: rkirby@theprostatecentre.com

Evangelos Liatsikos

Department of Urology, University of Patras, Patras, Greece

Alistair McGuire

LSE Health and Social Care, London School of Economics and Political Science, London, UK
e-mail: a.j.mcguire@lse.ac.uk

Declan G. Murphy

Department of Urology, Guy's & St Thomas' NHS Foundation Trust, London; Department of Urology, Royal Melbourne Hospital, Victoria, Australia
e-mail: decmurphy@doctors.net.uk

Imran Mushtaq

Great Ormond Street Hospital for Sick Children, London, UK
e-mail: imran.mushtaq@gstt.nhs.uk

Vipul R. Patel

Department of Robotic & Minimally Invasive Urologic Surgery, Florida Hospital Global Robotics Institute, Celebration, FL, USA
e-mail: vipul.patel.md@flhosp.org

Kenneth J. Palmer

Department of Urology, University of Miami, Coral Gables, FL, USA

Andreas John Papadopoulos

Department of Gynecologic Oncology, Maidstone Hospital, Maidstone, UK
e-mail: a.papadopoulos@nhs.net

Kankipati Shanti Raju

Department of Gynecologic Oncology, St Thomas' Hospital, London, UK
e-mail: shanti.raju@gstt.nhs.uk

P. Rimington
East Sussex Hospitals, Eastbourne, UK
e-mail: Peter.Rimington@esht.nhs.uk

Iqbal S. Shergill
St Bartholomews & the Royal London Hospitals, London, UK
e-mail: Super_iqi@yahoo.co.uk

Marcin Sicinski
Department of Anesthetics, Guy's & St Thomas' NHS Foundation Trust, London, UK
e-mail: marcin.scinski@gstt.nhs.uk

Dan Stoianovici
Department of URobotics, Johns Hopkins Hospital, Baltimore, MD, USA
e-mail: dss@jhu.edu

Jens-Uwe Stolzenburg
Department of Clinical Andrology, University of Leipzig, Leipzig, Germany

Qing Wang
Department of General Practice and Primary Care, School of Medicine, Kings College London, London, UK
e-mail: qing.wang@kcl.ac.uk

Chapter 1
Robotic Technology

Oussama Elhage and Nicholas Hegarty

> Any sufficiently advanced technology is indistinguishable
> from magic
> *Arthur C Clarke*

Abstract: Robotic surgery is an evolving and exciting field. We discuss the history of robotics in general and its introduction into medicine. Specific details of robotics in urology then follow with an introduction to the available systems. The chapter then concentrates on the da Vinci system which is currently the unchallenged master-slave platform. Comparisons between first and second generations of the da Vinci robot are made and improvements such as the 3DHD vision and Tile Pro are highlighted. Finally, there is a brief overview of telerobotics and telemedicine and a glimpse into the future of nanorobotics.

Keywords: Surgery, Technology, Robotic, Zeus, da Vinci

1.1. Introduction

Robotics in medicine in general and specifically in surgery is becoming an integral part of modern medical practice. All current indices suggest that this involvement will only increase. Here we briefly look at the history of robotics in surgery, discuss the various aspects of current systems, and explore other applications including telerobotics,

P. Dasgupta (ed.), *Robotic Urological Surgery in Clinical Practice*, 1
DOI: 10.1007/978-1-84800-243-2_1,
© Springer-Verlag London Limited 2008

telementoring, and virtual reality. We will finally provide a glimpse into the future of robotics in surgery.

1.2. Overview of Robotic Systems Development

1.2.1. History of Robotic Technology

Humans have used machines to facilitate the performance of difficult or mundane tasks from as early as 4000 B.C. Robots, on the other hand, were designed initially for entertainment. In the 4th century B.C. Archytas constructed the *pigeon*; the wings of this wooden bird were steam-driven allowing it to fly a distance of 200 m. Al-Jazari described automatic water-powered devices in the 11th century. One of these devices was a boat with musicians on board. Water-powered siphon mechanisms brought about arm movements playing flute, tambourine and harp, with the whistling of the flute being produced by water emptying through a tube (Donald 1974). Leonardo da Vinci was intrigued by mechanics and automation, developing a number of mannequins including a mechanical knight, bird, and lion. The lion was able to walk, stand up on its hind legs and present a bouquet of lilies to the king of France (Rosheim 2006). The "steam-man" was a design of the industrial age. It was a steam powered machine in the shape of a walking man which could pull a cart. Its torso formed the boiler and its bowler hat formed the chimney. It was first demonstrated in 1868 in New Jersey. This design inspired a series of stories published at the time in *Beadle's Dime Novels* about a man seeking adventures in the Wild West accompanied by a steam man (Nocks 2007).

Functional robotics, however, is a product of the twentieth and twenty-first centuries. The earlier models were designed to replicate human upper limb movements. In 1954 Devol developed a robotic arm which had an electronic feedback controller. Arm movements were programmable and driven by hydraulics. It was named Universal Automation which was later shortened to Unimation. The ability of the arm to slow its movement when approaching fixed objects was a major advance compared to previous models as well as the ability to perform multiple sequential tasks. Practical application was soon found in the assembly lines of General Motors plants, where it was used to handle hot metal for die-casting components of cars (Fig. 1.1). Extension of its role in industry beyond this however, took almost two decades. Further improvement came from Scheinman who designed the Stanford Arm at Stanford University. Compared to previous designs this model was lighter; the arm had a greater range of movement, was electrically rather than hydraulically powered, and it was able to perform more complex tasks. The commercially produced model was called: Programmable Universal Manipulation Arm (PUMA). This was the first truly flexible industrial robot and very soon became the

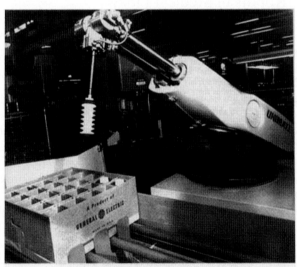

Armed for duty. A Unimate robot—really, just an arm— picks up and puts down parts in a General Electric factory.

FIGURE 1.1. Unimate, the first industrial robot, in a production line (Courtesy of: Robot Hall of Fame, Carnegie Mellon University).

industry standard. The ability to faithfully reproduce precise movements generated tremendous enthusiasm towards robotics in industry.

Mobility and broader functionality have been attributes of many of the more recently developed robots. Mobility (Cart, Genghis, Shadow Biped) with the ability to climb stairs and carry loads (Honda's Asimo), play music (Partner), provide companionship (Wakamaru, Nuvo), or provide pet simulation (Aibo, iCybie) are some of the functions performed by modern purpose-built robots. Others have been designed to collect specimens from outer space (Sojourner in the Mars Pathfinder mission), help assemble the international space station (SSRMS), and search for and rescue survivors at Ground Zero (Nocks 2007). Healthcare has also provided ample opportunity for the design and application of robotics.

1.3. Robots in Medical Fields

Medical and surgical robots still reflect the Czech origin of the name "*robota*" (forced labor) (Capek 1920). They can be divided into two large groups:

Robots in contact with patients: Assistive robots are designed to help those with restricted mobility or the elderly. Automatic guided wheelchairs consist of electric wheelchairs fitted with a processor and sensors and are designed to obey various commands to navigate indoors or outdoors (e.g., Wheelesley, SmartChair). Nursebot is designed to help the elderly: it reminds patients to take medicine, and can provide a consultation with a doctor through telepresence (Yanco 1998; Rao et al. 2002; Pineau et al. 2003). The RP-6 robot (InTouch Health, Santa Barbara, California) replaces the doctor at the bed side visit. The doctor is able to communicate with the patients through a wireless internet connection (Ellison et al. 2004). Rehabilitative robots help neurologically disabled patients to retrain the affected limb (Locomat) (Colombo et al. 2000). Surgical robots also fall into this category and are described later.

Other types of medical robots: These robots are used in the healthcare environment but not in direct contact with patients. They include transport robots and laboratory robots. Mobile robots carry specimens to the lab, some are designed to follow a predetermined route (lines on the floor) and some are able to navigate independently (Lob 1990; Prasad 1995). There are a wide variety of laboratory robots. Pipetting Station is an early design and is used in liquid handling and sampling. Cylindrical robots are designed to perform more complex tasks such as blood or HLA typing (Felder et al. 1990). Subsequently articulating robots were developed, being particularly useful in initial sorting and processing of samples. Sasaki from Japan integrated transport mobile robots with automated workstations realizing the concept of total laboratory automation. The human interface with the laboratory was only at final verification of results. He found that this system required one tenth the number of laboratory technicians previously used to serve a 600-bed hospital (Sasaki et al. 1998). Another development is near-patient unmanned remote laboratories which were developed at the University of Virginia (Boyd 2002) and can provide automated blood processing capabilities in an ambulatory setting. This concept is becoming more feasible as the size of laboratory equipment decreases, and new generations of handheld devices have begun to appear. The pharmaceutical industry has been quick to embrace robotics as its cost-effectiveness has become recognized in research and production laboratories. It has been found to be particularly useful in screening new molecules for the development of novel treatments.

1.4. Surgical Robots

The relative fixity of the cranium and skeleton were exploited to provide a platform for planning and execution of surgical procedures using early surgical robots in the fields of orthopaedics and neurosurgery. The Robodoc [Integrated

Surgical Systems Inc. (ISS), Davis, California] system was developed in the 1980s to perform hip replacements. It used the Orthodoc computer system for preoperative planning based on computed tomography (CT) imaging. During the operation itself the robotic arm equipped with a milling device was able to shape the desired cavity in the femur autonomously, though the process could be terminated by the surgeon in case of emergency (Bargar et al. 1998). The Caspar system was subsequently introduced using a similar approach. Both systems have, however, since been discontinued. An advance on these has been the Acrobot (The Acrobot Company, London, UK) which again uses preoperative radiographic imaging (X-ray and CT reconstructed images) to plan in relation to fixed operative site reference points. The software then plans the position of the prosthesis and cutting angles of the bones defining the proposed operative space. The robotic arms are subsequently manipulated by the surgeon to cut the preplanned planes within the restricted space employing the concept of "active constraint" (Jakopec et al. 2001). Though operatively precise, the extensive preoperative planning remains time consuming, limiting the appeal of this device. In neurosurgery the Unimation Puma 200 was introduced for brain biopsy and subsequently for a number of other procedures in the 1990s. A preoperative CT scan was used as a frame of reference. The coordinates of the lesion were programmed into the robot computer which then calculated the possible trajectories to the target area (biopsy or resection). The surgeon chose the optimum approach and executed the task using the robotic arm. NeuroMate™ (ISS, Davis, California) was another system developed in the same period and was used for stereotactic functional brain procedures. The early frame model was updated to a frameless one (Li et al. 2002). It was quite similar to Robodoc with both relying on image-guided preoperative planning. A later model of Minerva was able to provide CT guidance in real time so neurosurgical tools could be seen on images and alterations could be made in a dynamic fashion (Glauser et al. 1995). But this meant the patient has to be in the CT suite which was not practical. Other newer systems have been developed, the Pathfinder™ (Prosurgix, UK) (Eljamel 2007) with improved accuracy, and Cyberknife (Accuray, California) which was developed to deliver radiation therapy to malignant brain lesions and subsequently other malignancies using image guidance (Adler et al. 1999). The Cyberknife consists of two components: a targeting system and a mechanism to deliver high-dose radiation. The targeting system combines the pre-operative CT images with real-time intraoperative X-ray, and uses image-to-image correlation techniques to calculate and compensate automatically for target movements, realigning the beam to maintain a high level of accuracy (Chang et al. 2003). Cyberknife has the benefit of being less invasive than open surgical approaches, can target otherwise inaccessible lesions and do this with an accuracy to rival the most skilled of surgeons.

1.4.1. Robots in Urology

1.4.1.1. Various Designs

In urology, as in neurosurgery, the first robot to be used was a modified Unimation Puma 200. In the late 1980s a team from London led by Wickham combined the Puma model with a modified resectoscope and called it the Probot (Davies et al. 1989); they used it to perform transurethral resection of the prostate (TURP). It had a U-shaped frame to which the robot was attached with four axes of movement (in–out, rotation, tilt, and extension–retraction of the cutting element of the endoscope). The design allowed the endoscope to resect the prostate in a cone shape and restrict any movement beyond it. The endoscope had a liquidizer and an aspirator. Preoperative imaging was initially done by means of a transrectal ultrasound scan to determine the prostatic volume, but later used real-time transurethral scans (Harris et al. 1997). Though capable of autonomous resection of the prostate, completion of resection and hemostasis were still required to be performed by the surgeon with a manually operated endoscope. This limited the appeal of this system and its further development. Others have developed similar systems using lasers for prostate resection (Ho et al. 2001), but these too have failed to be adopted by urologists.

The next development was in prostate biopsies and renal access robots. A group from Milan used the SR 8438 Sankyo Scara "pick and place" robot to perform prostatic biopsies. They used transrectal ultrasound imaging for preoperative planning (Rovetta and Sala 1995). Further projects in robotic percutaneous needle access were developed. At Johns Hopkins, Baltimore, the Urobotics group developed the AcuBot. It consists of the PAKY-RCM (percutaneous access to the kidney-remote center of motion) and bridge mount and positioning platform designed for image-guided (fluoroscopy, CT) needle access. The PAKY-RCM component can be controlled by the surgeon using a joystick to manipulate the end-effector (needle) to a desired position. The arm is first passively fixed in position at the point of skin entry. Then by mimicking the surgical technique of aligning the needle entry point and needle target (renal calyx), the robotic system orientates the needle and registers the trajectory. The surgeon then moves the C-arm to the lateral view and by using a joystick is able to insert the needle to the desired depth (Stoianovici et al. 2003) (Fig. 1.2). This system can be used for needle biopsies, cryotherapy, and radiofrequency ablation. In a new project the same group has developed a magnetic resonance imaging (MRI) compatible robot called MrBot designed for brachytherapy seed implantations. The robot consists of two main elements: the controller unit (the computer and motion-control elements), and the MRI-compatible element which is made of ceramics, plastic and rubber materials, and operated by a specifically designed pneumatic motor. Initial in-vitro testing showed accurate seed placements (Muntener et al. 2006).

In the 1990s the Automated Endoscopic System for Optimum Positioning (AESOP) 1000 (Computer Motions,

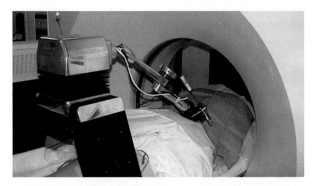

FIGURE 1.2. AcuBot surgical system with CT image guidance (Courtesy of: Dan Stoianovici).

Berkeley, California) was introduced to control laparoscopic instruments (camera and retractor). It consisted of a robotic arm controlled by a pedal. AESOP 2000 had voice control that responded to 23 commands. The current version is the AESOP 3000 and AESOP HR allows the surgeon to control it in addition to other devices in the operating room. AESOP provides steadier images than a human assistant, and allows solo surgery (Kavoussi et al. 1995; Kasalicky et al. 2002). A similar camera control system, the EndoAssist (Armstrong Healthcare, High Wycombe, UK), uses infrared technology.

1.4.1.2. Master–Slave Systems

Although some of the previously mentioned devices are master–slave robotic systems, where the robot is not autonomous and is manipulated by the surgeon, more advanced systems have since been developed. The Zeus (Computer Motions, California, subsequently Intuitive Surgical, Sunnyvale, California) combined the AESOP with two robotic manipulator arms attached separately by the patient side. The surgeon sat at the master console remote from the operating table. 3D vision was possible with polarizing glasses. The Zeus System was used in the first transatlantic

da Vinci® Surgical System in a Urology Procedure Setting

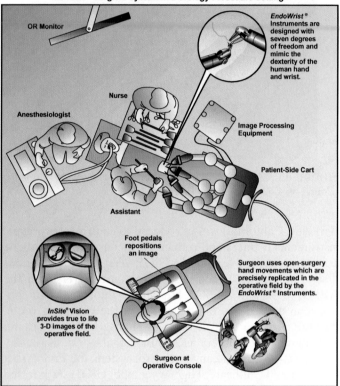

FIGURE 1.3. da Vinci master–slave system components (Courtesy of: Intuitive Surgical).

cholecystectomy in 2001 (Marescaux et al. 2001). Currently, the unchallenged master–slave system is the da Vinci™, developed by Intuitive Surgical, Sunnyvale, California.

The da Vinci™ system has three components (Fig. 1.3):

1. Surgeon's console.
2. Patient side cart.
3. Vision system.

Surgeon's console: This is a large unit where the surgeon sits remote from the patient. The unit contains the main computer, the hand controls which are operated by thumb and index fingers, a control panel and foot pedals for cautery, camera control, and clutching. The control panel provides the main system switch, emergency stop button, and other basic controls. The surgeon sits putting his head in the view ports and resting his forearms on the handle bar to use the hand controls. Intuitive movements at the handles are translated to the instruments at the patient's side. Motion scaling is possible with three options 1:1, 1:3, and 1:5. The most commonly used scaling in urology is 1:3 which means for every 3 cm movement of the surgeon's hand at the console there is translation of 1 cm movement at the operation site. 1:5 is commonly used in pediatric surgery. Vision is provided in 3D from two cameras with x10 magnification. The surgeon feels immersed in the operating field.

Patient side cart: This is the heaviest of the three. It consists of a central pole to which the robotic arms are mounted. The arms are first passively controlled and attached to trocars by the surgical assistants, this maneuver is called docking. The arm rotates around a fixed pivotal point marked on the cannula. One port is for the endoscope which has a light source and two high-resolution cameras (Fig. 1.4), the endoscope operates either at 0° or 30°. Two or three other ports are used for the specialized robotic instruments. These EndoWrist instruments have maneuverability comparable to that of a human wrist.

Vision system: This comprises two camera-control units which provide the 3D vision at the surgical console and a monitor which provides a 2D display for the assistants. A sound system is used for the surgeon to communicate with the assistants and vice versa. Other equipment includes a video recording device, a gas insufflator, and a light source.

The master console is connected to the surgical cart via a set of cables. The imaging stack is connected to the console via composite video and audio connector cables. The console

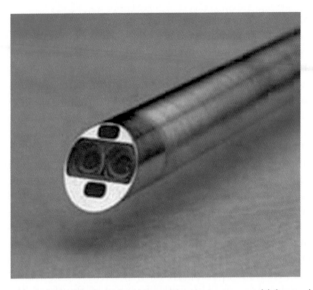

FIGURE 1.4. da Vinci endoscope with two cameras which provide the 3D vision at surgical console (Courtesy of: Intuitive Surgical).

has a battery that allows the system to keep functioning in case of a sudden loss of power.

The da Vinci™ system's popularity is multifactorial. This is a robotic system which allows the surgeon full control of the operative field mimicking conventional laparoscopy. It has the advantage of "intuition" where the instruments move in the same direction as the surgeon's hand, unlike laparoscopy where the surgeon has to adapt to the fulcrum effect at the abdominal wall where movement of the handle is translated to movement in the opposite direction at the effector site. The robotic instruments allow, in addition to motion scaling, steady, smooth, and precise movements eliminating the natural tremor of the human hand. The disadvantage is lack of tactile feedback which is compensated for by the 3D magnified display of the operative field at the surgical console. The EndoWrist technology is the most important feature of this system. It has enhanced maneuverability especially when performing complex tasks such as suturing or accessing deep-seated operating sites like the pelvis.

Intuitive Surgical has introduced two upgrades to its original design which remains essentially unchanged. The first upgrade added a 4th arm to the surgical cart and the second, the S-HD, brought a smaller surgical cart with improved vision and additional features which are summarized in Table 1.1.

All the above features make da Vinci™ an impressive piece of technology; however its monopoly of the master–slave robotic industry has relative disadvantages, mainly the purchasing and running costs. Some of the advantages and disadvantages are summarized in Table 1.2. Open surgery retains complete tactile feedback whereas laparoscopy retains some, and laparoscopic surgeons learn to adapt as part of the laparoscopic skills. Robotic surgeons learn to rely completely on their visual clues, but the lack of the haptics remains one of the major drawbacks. It is, however, possible to measure the manipulation forces of an instrument handling soft tissue. A piezoelectric tactile sensor

TABLE 1.1. Comparison of different da Vinci systems

	Standard da Vinci	da Vinci 4th arm	da Vinci S HD
Patient side cart	Standard	Standard	Motorized, smaller
Arms	3	4	4
Vision	3D	3D	3D HD
Adaptors	Multiple use	Multiple use	Integrated with drapes for multiple use
Instruments	8 mm	8 mm	8 mm or 5 mm
Additional features	-	-	Touch screen scope configuration
	-	-	Patient info multi-input display

TABLE 1.2. Advantages and disadvantages of the da Vinci robotic surgical systems (Adapted from: Murphy et al. 2006)

Advantages	Three-dimensional visualization
	Enhanced degrees-of-freedom
	No fulcrum effect
	Motion scaling
	Elimination of tremor
	Reduced fatigue
	Ergonomic position
Disadvantages	Expensive capital and running cost
	No tactile feedback
	Reduced trainee experience
	Lengthy setup time

has been developed that can be mounted on a surgical grasper (Dargahi et al. 2000). Other researchers used fiber-optic sensors which convey different light signals in response to various degrees of applied mechanical pressure. The signals are decoded in an opto-electronic converter. This method is MRI-compatible and has been integrated into a NeuroArm (Sutherland et al. 2003). A different approach is to attempt to test the characteristics of an organ with a tumor, which has a different "feel" to normal tissue with a static (Wellman and Howe 1997) or dynamic indentation probe (Noonan et al. 2007).

1.5. Virtual Reality, Telerobotics, and Telementoring

The ability of the surgeon to operate from a distance is an appealing one to various disciplines. It could be useful where specialist surgical expertise is unavailable, for example in rural areas, on board combat ships, and in space stations. In the 1980s a team from the National Aeronautics and Space Administration (NASA) working on Virtual Reality (VR) systems collaborated with Philip Green from the Stanford Research Institute (SRI) to develop the telepresence concept which is the basis for telerobotics (Satava 2002). The two main applications are:

- Telementoring.
- Telerobotic surgery.

Telementoring is guidance from a distance via visual and audio display devices. In surgery, the level of interaction varies between simple verbal guidance to control of laparoscopic instruments (telescope, retractors) via a robotic arm. An early experiment was reported from Johns Hopkins Hospital, Baltimore in 1996 where an experienced surgeon mentored another from 300 meters away during 23 cases. The mentor had control over an AESOP arm from a nearby operating room (Moore et al. 1996). The operative time was similar for simple procedures but longer for complex ones which included laparoscopic heminephrectomy and bladder augmentation. Soon after, aboard a US battleship in the Pacific Ocean, five inguinal hernia repairs were telementored from Maryland using the ship-to-shore satellite communication system (Cubano et al. 1999). A team from Yale University used a telephone modem with low bandwidth connection (12 kbps) to mentor operations in Ecuador (Rosser et al. 1999). The group from Johns Hopkins Hospital further developed their international telementoring program with several countries. This involved remote control of the AESOP and the PAKY-RCM robotic arms using high-speed telephone lines (Lee et al. 2000; Bove et al. 2003; Rodrigues et al. 2003).

Telerobotic surgery is when a surgeon operates from a distance using a robot. Rovetta et al. from Milan reported the first telerobotic procedure in 1995. Using their Sankyo SCA system which was mentioned earlier they performed a prostate biopsy; however, this was not developed further. The United States (US) Army took particular interest in the concept and developed a vehicle which has robotic arms manipulated by a distant surgeon. The wounded soldier would be put in the vehicle and the distant surgeon would perform just enough surgery to stop the hemorrhage prior to immediate transport to a more advanced surgical facility (Satava 2002). The first full telerobotic operation was performed by Prof. Marescaux in 2001. The surgeon in New York performed a robot-assisted laparoscopic cholecystectomy on a patient in France using the Zeus system (Marescaux et al. 2001). The connection was established via a Asynchronous Transfer Mode (ATM) network with a 10 Mb/s bandwidth for all data traffic with a time delay of 155 ms. A randomized controlled trial compared manual with robotic and transatlantic telerobotic percutaneous needle access into a kidney model. The transatlantic connection was between Guy's and Johns Hopkins Hospital via four Integrated Service Digital Network (ISDN) lines (Challacombe et al. 2003). The robotic-assisted insertions were slower, but more accurate and required fewer attempts compared to manual insertions.

The advancement in telecommunications is readily reflected in telemedicine. The availability of high-bandwidth connections allows reasonable quality of visual display and less time delay between the surgeon and operative site. The human mind can compensate for a time delay of up to 700 ms (Fabrizio et al. 2000). Despite its advantages, telerobotics remains expensive and has complicated ethical and medico-legal implications.

1.6. The Future

Current robotic technology is still developing and various concepts are being researched. Nanotechnology is emerging and expected to play an important role in diagnostics and minimally invasive treatment (Cavalcanti and Freitas 2005). The challenge is to manufacture nanodevices of carbon nanotubules and nanocrystals. Another challenge is data processing and storage. Nanodevices can be designed to deliver cancer drugs at cellular levels (Kawasaki and Player 2005). It is expected that future robotic devices will be smaller, cheaper, and more ergonomic. Eye-tracking to improve surgical vision and image-guided robotic surgery are just around the corner.

References

Adler JR Jr, Murphy MJ, Chang SD, Hancock SL (1999) Image-guided robotic radiosurgery. Neurosurgery 44:1299–1306

Bargar WL, Bauer A, Borner M (1998) Primary and revision total hip replacement using the Robodoc system. Clin Orthop Relat Res 82–91

Bove P, Stoianovici D, Micali S, Patriciu A, Grassi N, Jarrett TW, Vespasiani G, Kavoussi LR (2003) Is telesurgery a new reality? Our experience with laparoscopic and percutaneous procedures. J Endourol 17:137–142

Boyd J (2002) Tech Sight. Robotic laboratory automation. Science 295:517–518

Capek K (1920) Rossum's Universal Robots.

Cavalcanti A, Freitas RA Jr (2005) Nanorobotics control design: a collective behavior approach for medicine. IEEE Trans Nanobioscience 4:133–140

Challacombe BJ, Kavoussi LR, Dasgupta P (2003) Trans-oceanic telerobotic surgery. BJU Int 92:678–680

Chang SD, Main W, Martin DP, Gibbs IC, Heilbrun MP (2003) An analysis of the accuracy of the CyberKnife: a robotic frameless stereotactic radiosurgical system. Neurosurgery 52:140–146

Colombo G, Joerg M, Schreier R, Dietz V (2000) Treadmill training of paraplegic patients using a robotic orthosis. J Rehabil Res Dev 37:693–700

Cubano M, Poulose BK, Talamini MA, Stewart R, Antosek LE, Lentz R, Nibe R, Kutka MF, Mendoza-Sagaon M (1999) Long distance telementoring. A novel tool for laparoscopy aboard the USS Abraham Lincoln. Surg Endosc 13:673–678

Dargahi J, Parameswaran M, Payandeh S (2000) A micromachined piezoelectric tactile sensor for an endoscopic grasper-theory, fabrication, and experiments. J Microelectromech Syst 9:329

Davies BL, Hibberd RD, Coptcoat MJ, Wickham JE (1989) A surgeon robot prostatectomy—a laboratory evaluation. J Med Eng Technol 13:273–277

Donald H (1974) The Book of Knowledge of Ingenious Mechanical Devices. D. Reidel Publishing Company, Dordrecht

Eljamel MS (2007) Validation of the PathFinder™ neurosurgical robot using a phantom. Int J Med Robot 3(4):372–377

Ellison LM, Pinto PA, Kim F, Ong AM, Patriciu A, Stoianovici D, Rubin H, Jarrett T, Kavoussi LR (2004) Telerounding and patient satisfaction after surgery. J Am Coll Surg 199: 523–530

Fabrizio MD, Lee BR, Chan DY, Stoianovici D, Jarrett TW, Yang C, Kavoussi LR (2000) Effect of time delay on surgical performance during telesurgical manipulation. J Endourol 14: 133–138

Felder RA, Boyd JC, Margrey K, Holman W, Savory J (1990) Robotics in the medical laboratory. Clin Chem 36:1534–1543

Glauser D, Fankhauser H, Epitaux M, Hefti JL, Jaccottet A (1995) Neurosurgical robot Minerva: first results and current developments. J Image Guid Surg 1:266–272

Harris SJ, Arambula-Cosio F, Mei Q, Nathan MS, Hibberd RD, Wickham JE (1997) The Probot-an active robot for prostate resection. Proc Inst Mech Eng 211:317–325

Ho G, Ng WS, Teo MY, Kwoh CK, Cheng WS (2001) Experimental study of transurethral robotic laser resection of the prostate using the LaserTrode lightguide. J Biomed Opt 6:244–251

Marescaux J, Leroy J, Gagner M, Rubino F, Mutter D, Vix M et al. (2001) Transatlantic robot-assisted telesurgery. Nature 413: 379–380

Jakopec M, Harris SJ, Baena F, Gomes P, Cobb J, Davies BL (2001) The first clinical application of a "hands-on" robotic knee surgery system. Comput Aided Surg 6:329–339

Kasalicky MA, Svab J, Fried M, Melechovsky D (2002) AESOP 3000—computer-assisted surgery, personal experience. Rozhl Chir 81:346–349

Kavoussi LR, Moore RG, Adams JB, Partin AW (1995) Comparison of robotic versus human laparoscopic camera control. J Urol 154:2134–2136

Kawasaki ES, Player A (2005) Nanotechnology, nanomedicine, and the development of new, effective therapies for cancer. Nanomedicine 1:101–109

Lee BR, Png DJ, Liew L, Fabrizio M, Li MK, Jarrett JW, Kavoussi LR (2000) Laparoscopic telesurgery between the United States and Singapore. Ann Acad Med Singapore 29:665–668

Li QH, Zamorano L, Pandya A, Perez R, Gong J, Diaz F (2002) The application accuracy of the NeuroMate robot—A quantitative comparison with frameless and frame-based surgical localization systems. Comput Aided Surg 7:90–98

Lob WS (1990) Robotic transportation. Clin Chem 36:1544–1550

Moore RG, Adams JB, Partin AW, Docimo SG, Kavoussi LR (1996) Telementoring of laparoscopic procedures: initial clinical experience. Surg Endosc 10:107–110

Muntener M, Patriciu A, Petrisor D, Mazilu D, Bagga H, Kavoussi L, Cleary K, Stoianovici D (2006) Magnetic resonance imaging compatible robotic system for fully automated brachytherapy seed placement. Urology 68:1313–1317

Murphy D, Challacombe B, Khan MS, Dasgupta P (2006) Robotic technology in urology. Postgraduate Med J 82:743–747

Nocks L (2007) The robot: the life story of a technology. Greenwood Press, Westport

Noonan D, Liu H, Zweiri Y (2007) A dual-function wheeled probe for tissue viscoelastic property identification during minimally invasive surgery. In: Robotics and Automation, 2007 IEEE International Conference, April 10th–14th, 2007, Rome

Pineau J, Montemerlo M, Pollack M, Ray N, Thrun S (2003) Towards robotic assistants in nursing homes: Challenges and results. Robot Autonom Syst 42:271–281

Prasad P (1995) Effective use of robots as mechanized couriers at Stanford University Hospital. Biomed Instrum Technol 29:398–404

Rao RS, Conn K, Jung SH, Katupitiya J, Kientz T, Kumar V, Ostrowski J, Patel S, Taylor CJ (2002) Human robot interaction: Applications to smart wheelchairs. In: Robotics and Automation. Proc ICRA '02. IEEE International Conference, 11th–15th May, 2002

Rodrigues NN Jr, Mitre AI, Lima SV, Fugita OE, Lima ML, Stoianovici D, Patriciu A, Kavoussi LR (2003) Telementoring between Brazil and the United States: initial experience. J Endourol 17:217–220

Rosheim ME (2006) Leonardo's lost robots. Springer, Berlin Heidelberg New York

Rosser JC Jr, Bell RL, Harnett B, Rodas E, Murayama M, Merrell R (1999) Use of mobile low-bandwidth telemedical techniques for extreme telemedicine applications. J Am Coll Surg 189: 397–404

Rovetta A, Sala R (1995) Execution of robot-assisted biopsies within the clinical context. J Image Guid Surg 1:280–287

Sasaki M, Kageoka T, Ogura K, Kataoka H, Ueta T, Sugihara S (1998) Total laboratory automation in Japan. Past, present, and the future. Clin Chim Acta 278:217–227

Satava RM (2002) Surgical robotics: the early chronicles: a personal historical perspective. Surg Laparosc Endosc Percutan Tech 12:6–16

Stoianovici D, Cleary K, Patriciu A, Mazilu D, Stanimir A, Craciunoiu N, Watson V, Kavoussi L (2003) AcuBot: a Robot for radiological interventions. In: IEEE Transactions on Robotics and Automation, pp. 927–930

Sutherland G, McBeth P, Louw D (2003) NeuroArm: an MR compatible robot for microsurgery. Int Congress Series 1256:504

Wellman P, Howe R (1997) Modelling probe and tissue interaction for tumour feature extraction. In: ASME Summer Bioengineering Conference, Sun River, Oregon

Yanco H (1998) Wheelesley: A robotic Wheelchair System: Indoor Navigation and User Interface. In: Mittal VO (ed) Assistive Technology and Artificial Intelligence. Springer, Berlin Heidelberg New York, pp. 256–268

Chapter 2
The Basic Science of Robotic Surgery

Ben Challacombe and Dan Stoianovici

Abstract: This chapter aims to cover the basic science of robotic surgery focusing on all the devices currently in clinical use. We hope to give the potential and practicing robotic surgeon an understanding of the scientific basis behind the machines themselves and provide a concise framework of the practical nuances.

Keywords: Degrees of freedom, Remote centre of motion, Ergonomics

2.1. Introduction

The definition of the term robot would state that they are "mechanical devices that sometimes resemble human beings and are capable of performing a variety of complex human tasks on command, or by being programmed in advance." Robots as we know them today were developed after the Second World War due to the increased demand for automation in automobile production and worked on a few basic principles. However, the requirements of the surgical robots we use today, which are designed to be precise, accurate, and safe have little in common with these industrial robots which were characterized by their fast, strong, and repeatable actions. We

P. Dasgupta (ed.), *Robotic Urological Surgery in Clinical Practice*,
DOI: 10.1007/978-1-84800-243-2_2,
© Springer-Verlag London Limited 2008

look at some of the science behind the robotic devices themselves from an easy-to-use and clinical perspective.

2.2. Robotic Systems and Terminology

The robots used in surgery should ideally be part of a computer-integrated surgery system. The robot is just one element of a larger system designed to assist a surgeon in performing a surgical procedure (Cepolina et al. 2005).

Medical robots may be classified in many different ways: by manipulator design (e.g., kinematics, actuation, degrees-of-freedom) (Taylor and Stoianovici 2003); by their level of autonomy (e.g., preprogrammed, image-guided, teleoperated, synergetic); by the targeted anatomy/technique (e.g., cardiac, intravascular, percutaneous, laparoscopic, microsurgical); by the intended operating environment (e.g., operating room, imaging scanner, hospital floor); or by context of their role in computer-integrated surgery systems (surgical planner, surgical assistants).

Surgical robots are required to work within properly structured constraints to ensure patient safety; however, the working environment cannot always be predicted and potentially dangerous situations can quickly develop. Thus, any changes in the robot's environment need to be swiftly recognized and the crisis response and safe recovery autonomously initiated, with this information displayed to the surgeon, along with possible options for subsequent safe continued use. The proper setting of autonomous limitations is a subtle question, and adjustment to an individual surgeon's requirements or complete overriding must be possible.

From these general features, robotic surgery is seen to be a technology-driven development in two particular areas:

- Information infrastructure: data acquisition, handling, vaulting, transmission, validation, processing, etc. These are continuously expanding options supported by the

ICT (Information and Communications Technology), and effective new computer tools ceaselessly appear to support remote supervision and control. Telemedicine is a fully acknowledged technology, while remote surgery has already displayed some noteworthy accomplishments.

• Execution effectors: specialized tools and fixtures are the most challenging research subjects, which are continuously evolving to adapt to more precise and demanding performance.

In the future, surgeons will continue to use standard-sized tools, but the inner-body interface will continue to

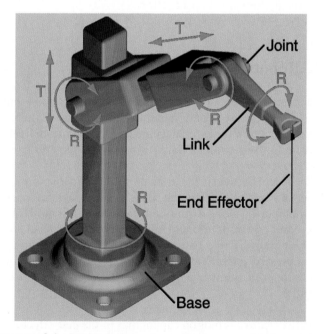

FIGURE 2.1. Basic design of a robotic arm showing potential movements/degrees-of-freedom about each joint (Courtesy of: URobotics Dept, Johns Hopkins University).

move towards micro and nanosurgery (Ebbesen and Jensen 2006) as soon as effective new technologies are commercially available.

With this in mind, an effective robotic surgical system should permit:

- Tactile feedback, to appreciate the compliance of human tissue;
- Kinesthetic restitution, to govern the grasping/handling forces;
- Three-dimensional (3D) vision to enable precise hand–eye co-ordination;
- Six degrees-of-freedom (DoF) (e.g., Fig. 2.1) to enable full dexterity for surgical procedures.

2.3. Robotic Movements

These need to be integrated into technical frames, built on: (1) end-effectors path/mobility redundancy; (2) intelligence for autonomous management; (3) operational reliability and intrinsic safety; and (4) in-process diagnostics and self-recovery.

Each joint within such a system must be capable of multi-planer movement to allow the robot to move with an acceptable number of DoF. A pin joint has one rotational DoF, a slider joint one translational DoF, and a ball and socket joint, three rotational DoF. Thus, any complex movement can be decompressed into its elementary motions. A robot's DoF equals the total number of joint DoF. These movements can be either

- Active: Conveys motion capabilities of the end-effector.
- Passive: Conveys prepositioning capabilities.

The number of active DoF also signifies the number of motors involved. Any DoF <6 will result in some restricted maneuverability whilst a DoF >6 may lead to redundant or occasionally enhanced movements.

2.4. Remote Center of Motion (RCM)

The RCM is a key concept in surgical robotics. It consists of a fulcrum point that is located distal to the mechanism itself, typically at the skin entry point/laparoscopic port site in percutaneous devices. This allows the RCM to precisely orientate a surgical instrument/needle in space while maintaining the needle tip at the skin entry point (or another specified location) without placing unwanted traction or pressure on this point. Initially the RCM concept was developed in percutaneous robots such as the PAKY-RCM (Fig. 2.2). This robot consisted of a seven DOF lockable manipulator, or passive

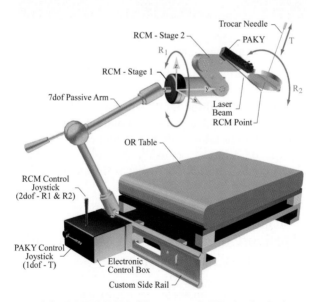

FIGURE 2.2. PAKY-RCM (Courtesy of: URobotics Laboratory, Johns Hopkins University).

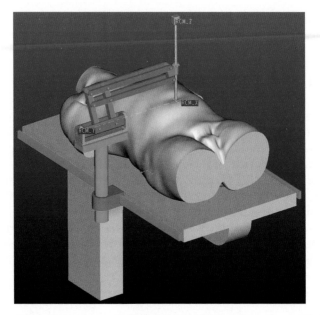

FIGURE 2.3. Laparoscopic RCM device. This has four external DoF (three rotational and one translational).

arm, connected to a three DOF active arm. The arm houses a radiolucent needle driver and is mounted using a side rail onto the operating table. Current examples of RCM robots include the da Vinci™, Zeus™, Aesop™, and Acubot® devices. A laparoscopic RCM device is shown in Fig. 2.3.

2.5. Surgical Computer-Aided Design/Computer-Aided Manufacturing Systems (CAD/CAM)

CAD/CAM systems transform preoperative images and other clinical information into models of individual patients. These models can be used to preplan intervention and test a variety of potential clinical scenarios. Intraoperatively, these data can be registered to the actual patient and used as an image overlay display to assist in the accurate execution of a planned intervention. The CAD/CAM systems can be incorporated with mechanical robotic devices to perform an actual intervention. Data from the model, as well as real-time patient data, are integrated and used to guide a needle, instrument, or probe into a desired target. Their purpose is to act as a trajectory-enforcement device, correctly aligning the end-effectors based on ultrasonography, fluoroscopy, CT, or MRI. These systems can perform a task defined by the treating physician with great accuracy. By integrating preoperative planning and intraoperative decision-making, the potential exists for improved outcomes with minimal errors. Orthopedics and neurosurgery were the first fields to use these surgical CAD/CAM systems because their procedures involved well-defined, fixed anatomic landmarks that could be easily imaged.

In neurosurgery stereotactic frames were developed using the fixed landmarks of the rigid cranium. Neurosurgical stereotactic procedures with the robot (NeuroMate, Integrated Surgical Systems, Davis, California) (Benabid et al. 1992) positioning the needle guides in predefined targets and hip replacement surgeries with the robot (Robodoc, Integrated Surgical Systems) milling a cavity to exactly fit the implant are examples of CAD/CAM surgical systems (Paul et al. 1992).

It has been more challenging to develop similar systems in soft-tissue specialties. The first such autonomous system in clinical use in urology was the Probot in 1989 (Davies et al. 1989, 1991). This was a joint venture between Guy's Hospital and the Mechanical Engineering Department Imperial College, London and the device was built to perform transurethral resection of the prostate (TURP). The relatively fixed position of the prostate and the repetitive motions involved in a TURP made this an attractive candidate for robotic CAD/CAM assistance. The mechanical system used a standard resectoscope mounted on a stereotactic frame. The system used video and ultrasound information and the surgeon predefined the desired resection area according to the

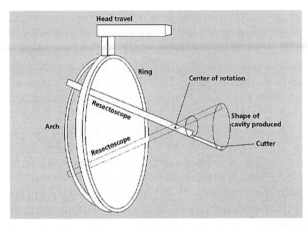

FIGURE 2.4. The Wickham TUR frame (Courtesy of: J Wickham and S Nathan).

ultrasound images. The robot then resected as instructed and did so in an efficient manner. Drawbacks such as the inaccuracy of transrectal ultrasonography in determining prostate dimensions, as well as the need for manual chip removal and hemostasis, prevented further adoption into clinical practice. An example of a TUR frame is given in Fig. 2.4.

2.6. Percutaneous Renal Access

Percutaneous access to the renal collecting system for nephrolithotomy has also been a focus of attention for CAD/CAM systems. Dan Stoianovici from Johns Hopkins University designed, built, and clinically trialed the RCM (Fig. 2.5) and percutaneous access to the kidney (PAKY) devices (Su et al. 2002). The system is able to perform fully automated needle placements in soft tissues. As discussed the RCM is a general-purpose module for robotic procedures whilst the PAKY is a needle driver module. The robot is compact (171 × 69 × 52 mm box) and weighs only 1.6 kg

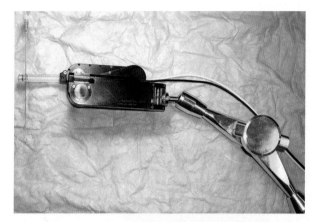

FIGURE 2.5. The RCM robot (Courtesy of: URobotics Laboratory, Johns Hopkins University).

facilitating its placement within an imaging device. It consists of a fulcrum point that is located distal to the mechanism itself, typically at the skin entry point. This allows the RCM to precisely orientate a needle in space while maintaining the needle tip at the skin entry point (Varkarakis et al. 2005).

In contrast to the earlier LARS robot (Cadeddu et al. 1997) the RCM (e.g., Fig. 2.6) employs a chain transmission rather than a parallel linkage. This permits unrestricted rotations about the RCM point, uniform rigidity of the mechanism, and eliminates singular points. The needle is initially placed into the PAKY such that its tip is located at the remote center of motion. To confirm the position the PAKY is equipped with a visible laser diode whose ray intersects the needle at the RCM point. The robot permits two motorized DoF about the RCM point.

The fulcrum point is located distal to the mechanism itself; the needle can translate and rotate while preserving the position of its insertion point. Overall, the system has ten DoF: seven passive DoF are used to orient and position the arm that sustains the RCM. The RCM has two active rotational DoF for positioning the needle inside the patient; PAKY has

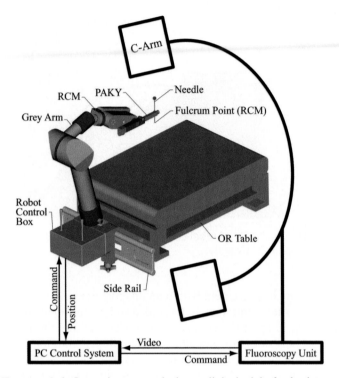

FIGURE 2.6. Operative set up during a clinical trial of robotic percutaneous access.

one active DoF for driving the needle. In comparison with traditional techniques, the robot is able to reduce tremor, minimize radiation exposure, and increase accuracy; the error is circa. 1 mm. The needle, an inexpensive sterile disposable part, is radiolucent to allow real time-control, and an electrical bioimpedance sensor provides the needle-force feedback (Hernandez et al. 2001). If being used for PCNL, the urologist selects the target calyx and provides this information to the robot, which then performs the task of placing the needle in the predefined point. Johns Hopkins developed a system with these features using an active robot and biplanar fluoroscopy. In a manner similar to extracorporeal lithotripsy, the surgeon selected the target calyx on two images and the robot inserted the needle into the desired location (Stoianovici et al. 2003). However, it also revealed several problems related to the respiratory mobility and deformability of the kidney, which were considered responsible for the 50% success rate on first attempt. Guy's Hospital, London, and Johns Hopkins University have collaborated and conducted a randomized controlled trial of locally and transatlantic robotically assisted percutaneous needle insertions, showing the PAKY-RCM robot to be more accurate than the human hand but slightly slower. The time and accuracy of robotic teleoperations are similar to those of locally aided robotic interventions (Challacombe et al. 2005).

2.7. Telesurgery

Telesurgery is performed between a primary operating theatre and a remotely located control room. Both sites should be connected with high bandwidth communication lines over which audiovisual (teleconferencing) and motion data (robot control) will be transmitted. The remote control room should be equipped with the following: (a) a high-resolution video monitor allowing for simultaneous presentation of both external and internal operating video images from the primary operating site; (b) a multidirectional microphone and speaker to allow communication between the remote and primary surgeons; (c) a robotic control console, haptic interface, or even a control pad to allow the remote surgeon to control the remotely located robotic device (e.g., AESOP, electrocautery); and (d) a telestrator video sketchpad, which may be very instrumental for the remote surgeon to illustrate the operative plan to the local team. Similarly, the persons in the primary operating suite should be able to see and listen to the remote instructor with the help of similar audiovisual media (video, microphone, and speaker). An additional external camera coupled with a motor to pan and tilt when controlled from the remote site will transmit images of what is happening in the distant operating room. Finally, the purposely built robotic device should be located near the patient in the operating suite and remotely controlled from the distant control room. Delays in the transmission of information must be less than 300 ms (Janetschek et al. 1998) otherwise remote task performance will be significantly hindered. For transport of the high number of audio, video, and medical images required during telesurgery, dedicated asynchronous transfer mode (ATM) lines are considered the most reliable and safe. Communication delays are dependent on the distance between the sites, but previous experience (Lee et al. 1998, 2000) (delays of only up to 155 ms) and speed calculations have shown that these delays are acceptable when performing earth-to-earth connections.

Telementoring in urology has been pioneered by the Baltimore group who have telementored several procedures in Austria, Singapore, Italy, Germany including laparoscopic adrenalectomy, radical nephrectomy, varicocelectomy, renal cyst ablation, and PCNL (Bauer et al. 2001; Bove et al. 2003). Telerobotic control was achieved via ISDN lines. Internet connections are generally currently favored and are cheaper. The fastest but most expensive telelinks use satellite connections. The concept of having a surgeon in one country performing an operation in another via a computer-assisted link became reality in 2001 when a laparoscopic cholecystectomy was performed on a patient in Strasbourg by a surgeon in New York using the Zeus telerobotic system (Lindbergh Operation) (Marescaux et al. 2001). French telecom provided high-speed ATM lines for this landmark procedure. As illustrated in other telesurgical trials time delay can significantly affect surgical performance; however if the lag time is <700 ms the surgeon is able to learn to compensate (Fabrizio et al. 2000).

The PAKY-RCM arm has also been used as the first step in transcontinental (e.g., Fig. 2.7) PCNL between two countries albeit in only a few patients (Bauer et al. 2001; Rodrigues et al. 2003). It has been adapted for use in percutaneous biopsies with CT guidance. For targeting purposes CT guidance has the advantage of using potentially automated

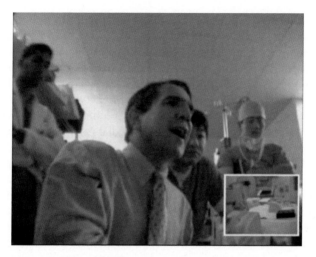

FIGURE 2.7. STAR TRAK~ Systematic Trans Atlantic Randomized Tele Robotic Access to the Kidney. The *inset* shows telerobotic PCNL being performed over high-speed lines with real time robotic, voice, image, and fluoroscopic control.

guidance and thus reduces the level of expertise required to successfully and repeatedly perform percutaneous access. Initial clinical trials on 16 patients were successful for all interventional procedures including ten percutaneous core biopsies, a nephrostomy tube placement and a neobladder access (Solomon et al. 2002). Needle readjustment was required in four cases that required a second pass. This system has now been integrated with CT scanning and used in clinical trials.

2.8. Multi-Imager Compatible Actuation Principles in Surgical Robotics

It is felt that today's robots have not achieved their full potential. One way forward is to integrate them with real-time image guidance which is a concept that is currently being developed. However, imager compatibility raises significant engineering challenges for robotic systems. Although the majority of robotic components may be redesigned with MRI-compatible materials, the electromagnetic motors most commonly used in robotic actuation are incompatible. The Hopkins URobotics group has described two new types of pneumatic/hydraulic motors that may enable the development of better performance image-guided robots (Stoianovici et al. 2007a).

MrBot is the first robot for fully-automated image-guided access of the prostate gland (Fig. 2.8). The robot is customized for transperineal needle insertion and designed to be compatible with all known types of medical-imaging equipment. This includes uncompromised compatibility with magnetic resonance imagers (MRI) of the highest field strength, size accessibility within closed-bore tunnel-shaped scanners, and clinical intervention safety. The robot is designed to accommodate various end-effectors for different percutaneous interventions such as biopsy, serum injections, or

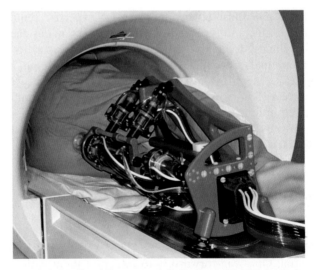

FIGURE 2.8. Mr Bot (Courtesy of: D Stoianovici, URobotics).

brachytherapy. For MRI compatibility the robot is exclusively constructed from nonmagnetic and dielectric materials such as plastics, ceramics, and rubbers and is electricity free. The system utilizes a new type of motor specifically designed for this application, the pneumatic stepper motor (PneuStep). These uniquely provide easily controllable precise and safe pneumatic actuation. Fiber-optical encoding is used for feedback, so that all electric components are distally located outside the imager's room (Stoianovici et al. 2007b).

2.9. Ergonomics

The arrival of complex master–slave robotic systems in the operating theatre may help resolve some of the ergonomic obstacles facing minimally invasive surgeons. These include eye-strain and the large movements outside the patient which cause arm and neck pain among laparoscopic surgeons. In addition the pistol-type handles force the hands into extreme positions of flexion and ulnar deviation at the wrist which require more muscle contractions to perform a task compared with in-line handle or open techniques (Elhage et al. 2007). The cumulative effect of the problems listed above is to increase overall fatigue and stress and restrict the number of MIS procedures that can be performed by one surgeon in a given operative session.

The da Vinci S^{TM} system (Intuitive Surgical, Sunnyvale, California) is the most-advanced "robotic" system currently available. Having the surgeon seated at a console remote from the patient provides a much more ergonomic posture than that of the traditional patient-side surgeon. The fingertip controls allow "intuitive" rather than "fulcrum"-type control over the laparoscopic instruments, thereby reducing fatigue in the upper extremity and neck. The restoration of seven DoF compared with the four DoF of conventional laparoscopy seems to offer considerable benefits for complex laparoscopic tasks (Talamini et al. 2002). This should also decrease the excessive wrist strain during laparoscopy.

3D-stereoscopic vision can also provide advantages over the 2D-monoscopic vision of conventional laparoscopic systems (Jourdan et al. 2004). One mechanism of reducing surgeon fatigue in laparoscopic prostatectomy is to employ the AESOP robot as a camera holder and this is now standard practice in many units.

2.10. AESOP

The Automated Endoscopic System for Optimal Positioning (AESOP, Computer Motion, California) is a robotic arm designed to hold and manipulate a laparoscope. It is one of a number of auxiliary surgical-support systems, which work side-by-side with the surgeon and perform such functions as endoscope holding or retraction. The AESOP is affixed to the operating table, has six degrees-of-freedom, two of which are passive (meaning they are positioned by hand), and can be controlled with hand, foot, or voice control interface. This device is optimally voice controlled and the surgeon has a preprogrammed voice card that allows the machine to understand and respond to his or her commands. Laparoscopic images are steadier, with fewer camera changes and inadvertent instrument collisions than an inexperienced human assistant (Kavoussi et al. 1995).

2.11. The da Vinci™ Robot

Because of the intellectual property rights of Intuitive Surgical there is relatively little known about the intricate workings of the world's most popular and prevalent robotic system, the da Vinci™ robot (Figs. 2.9–2.11). However, the fundamental building block of surgical robotics is the robotic arm itself due to its unique position as the end-effector of robotic systems and in the da Vinci system this again follows basic robotic principles (Moran 2007). Amazingly, Leonardo da Vinci himself designed the first sophisticated robotic arm in

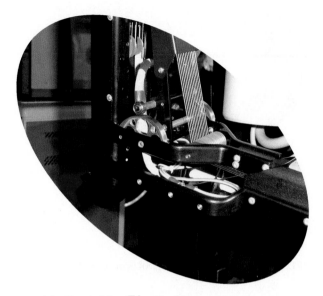

FIGURE 2.9. The da Vinci™ cable drive system.

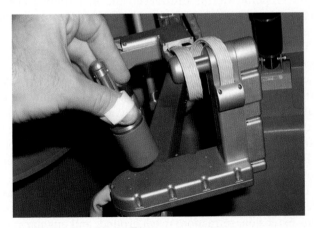

FIGURE 2.10. The da Vinci™ finger manipulators.

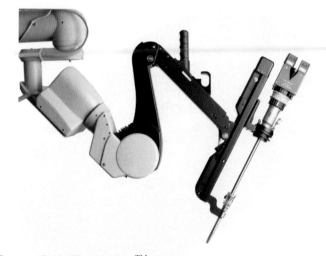

FIGURE 2.11. The da Vinci™ surgical arm (a RCM).

1495 with four degrees-of-freedom and an analogue on-board controller supplying power and programmability (Rosheim 2000). General Motors introduced the first robotic arm in 1962, the Unimate robot, invented by George Devol and marketed by Joseph Engelberger (Devol et al. 1961).

The system uses 3-D imaging to immerse the surgeon in a three-dimensional video operating field with 6–10x magnification. The modern da Vinci robot has a series of joints with the most robust (the shoulder) placed centrally by the central tower and the most delicate end-effectors (fingers or instruments) placed peripherally. Each joint has a set degree of freedom and a defined range of movement. The arm itself is an RCM system (see earlier) with a fixed range of movements about a skin entry point.

The shoulder joint bears the highest load but also has a large range of movement, with three DoF. The elbow provides extension, retraction, reach around, and angular reorientation of the wrist and hand. The wrist is the most vital joint and allows the end-effectors (instruments) to be precisely manipulated in three-dimensional space. It is this joint which is truly the most indispensible constituent within the da Vinci system. However, like the human wrist, if articulated 45° off center, its ability to roll degenerates, resulting in joint locking. The hand is represented by the instruments themselves which are the end-effectors. Many feel that the lack of tactile feedback is compensated for by the excellent 3D optics.

2.12. Endowrist®

The Endowrist® is vital to the increased maneuverability possible with the da Vinci robotic system. The surgeon's forefinger and thumb motions are intuitively translated into movements of the robotic arms. Standard manual laparoscopy (Fig. 2.12) has five DoF (four external and one internal, i.e., grasping, cutting) whilst the addition of the Endowrist® (Fig. 2.13) permits an increase in DoF from five to seven (four external and three internal).

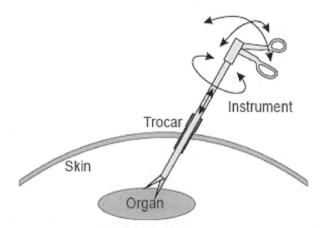

FIGURE 2.12. Four laparoscopic DoF (Courtesy of: Department of Mechanical Engineering, Katholieke Universiteit Leuven. http://www.mech.kuleuven.be/robotics/ras/).

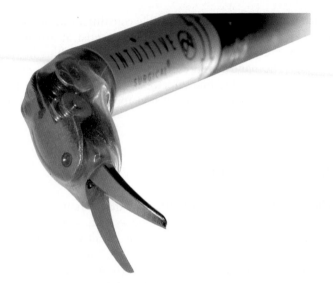

FIGURE 2.13. da Vinci Endowrist with three additional DoF.

2.13. The Future of Surgical Robotic Science

The da Vinci robot is unlikely to represent the ultimate robotic surgical system and it should be seen as the current most highly sophisticated master–slave system on a stepwise progression of robotic development. The devices themselves will become smaller, lighter, and integrated into telesurgical systems. This will allow the seamless integration of patient data and imaging into the robotic console permitting real-time intraoperative visualization of pathology and other tissues. This augmented reality surgery combining laparoscopic images with virtual 3D images will help identify and avoid injury to key structures. Instruments will continue to decrease in size to true needlescopic (2 mm) end-effectors and a haptic feedback system is likely to arrive within five years.

Other areas of development include the snake-like or serpentine robots which are now being targeted toward the field of natural orifice surgery. Known as NOTES™ (Natural Orifice Transluminal Endoscopic Surgery), these robots have multiple degrees-of-freedom, do not fail if one joint locks/blocks, and can be used transgastrically (Hochbergerand Lamade 2005). They open the door for external woundless/scarless surgery and procedures including cholecystectomies, appendicectomies, and tubal ligations have already occurred. A sound grasp of the basic robotic science behind the machines may prove vital to further surgical developments in this exciting field.

References

Bauer J, Lee BR, Stoianovici D et al. (2001) Remote percutaneous renal access using a new automated telesurgical robotic system. Telemed J E Health 7:341–346

Benabid AL, Lavallee S, Hoffmann D et al. (1992) Computer driven robot for stereotactic neurosurgery. In: Kelly PJ, Kall BA (eds) Computers in Stereotactic Neurosurgery. Boston, Blackwell, pp 330–342

Bove P, Stoianovici D, Micali S et al. (2003) Is telesurgery a new reality? Our experience with laparoscopic and percutaneous procedures. J Endourol 17:137–142

Cadeddu JA, Bzostek A, Schreiner S, Barnes AC, Roberts WW, Anderson JH et al. (1997) A robotic system for percutaneous renal access. J Urol 158:1589–1593

Cepolina F, Challacombe B, Michelini RC (2005) Trends in robotic surgery. J Endourol 19:940–951

Challacombe B, Patriciu A, Glass J, Aron M, Jarrett T, Kim F et al. (2005) A randomized controlled trial of human versus robotic and telerobotic access to the kidney as the first step in percutaneous nephrolithotomy. Comput Aided Surg 10(3):165–171

Davies BL, Hibberd RD, Coptcoat MJ et al. (1989) A surgeon robot prostatectomy—a laboratory evaluation. J Med Eng Technol 13:273–277

Davies BL, Hibberd RD, Ng WS et al. (1991) The development of a surgeon robot for prostatectomies. Proc Inst Mech Eng 205:35–38

Devol G (1961) US Patent 2,988,237. Programmed article transfer. Filed December 10, 1954 and issued June 13, 1961

Ebbesen M, Jensen TG (2006) Nanomedicine: techniques, potentials, and ethical implications. J Biomed Biotechnol 5:51516

Elhage O, Murphy D, Challacombe B, Shortland A, Dasgupta P (2007) Ergonomics in minimally invasive surgery. Int J Clin Pract 61:186–188

Fabrizio MD, Lee BR, Chan DY, Stoianovici D, Jarrett TW, Yang C, Kavoussi LR (2000) Effect of time delay on surgical performance during telesurgical manipulation. J Endourol 14: 133–138

Hernandez DJ, Sinkov VA, Roberts WW, Allaf ME, Patriciu A, Jarrett TW et al. (2001) Measurement of bio-impedance with a smart needle to confirm percutaneous kidney access. J Urol 166(4):1520–1523

Hochberger J, Lamade W (2005) Transgastric surgery in the abdomen: the dawn of a new era? Gastrointest Endosc 62(2): 293–296

Janetschek G, Bartsch G, Kavoussi LR (1998) Transcontinental interactive laparoscopic telesurgery between the United States and Europe. J Urol 160:1413

Jourdan IC, Dutson E, Garcia A et al. (2004) Stereoscopic vision provides a significant advantage for precision robotic laparoscopy. Br J Surg 91:879–885

Kavoussi LR, Moore RG, Adams JB et al. (1995) Comparison of robotic versus laparoscopic camera control. J Urol 154: 2134–2136

Lee BR, Bishoff JT, Janetschek G et al. (1998) A novel method of surgical instruction: international telementoring. World J Urol 16:367–370

Lee BR, Png DJ, Liew L et al. (2000) Laparoscopic telesurgery between the United States and Singapore. Ann Acad Med Singapore 29:665–668

Marescaux J, Leroy J, Gagner M et al. (2001) Transatlantic robot-assisted telesurgery. Nature 413:379–380

Moran ME (2007) Evolution of robotic arms. J Robotic Surg 1: 103–111

Paul HA, Bargar WL, Mittlestadt B et al. (1992) Development of a surgical robot for cementless total hip arthroplasty. Clin Orthop 285:57–66

Rodrigues NN Jr, Mitre AI, Lima SV, Fugita OE, Lima ML, Stoianovici D et al. (2003) Telementoring between Brazil and the United States: Initial experience. J Endourol 17:217–220

Rosheim ME (2000) Leonardo's programmable automaton. A reconstruction. http://www.anthrobot.com/press/article_leo_programmable.html (last accessed 15.04.2008)

Solomon SB, Patriciu A, Bohlman ME, Kavoussi LR, Stoianovici D (2002) Robotically driven interventions: a method of using CT fluoroscopy without radiation exposure to the physician. Radiology 225:277–282

Stoianovici D, Cleary K, Patriciu A et al. (2003) AcuBot: A robot for radiological interventions. IEEE Trans Robotics Automation 19:926–930.

Stoianovici D, Patriciu A, Mazilu D, Petrisor D, Kavoussi L (2007a) A new type of motor: Pneumatic step motor. IEEE/ASME Transactions on Mechatronics 12:98–106

Stoianovici D, Song D, Petrisor D, Ursu D, Mazilu D, Muntener M et al. (2007b) "MRI stealth" robot for prostate interventions. Minim Invasiv Ther 16:241–248

Su LM, Stoianovici D, Jarrett TW et al. (2002) Robotic percutaneous access to the kidney: Comparison with standard manual access. J Endourol 16:471–475

Talamini M, Campbell K, Stanfield C (2002) Robotic gastrointestinal surgery: early experience and system description. J Laparoendosc Adv Surg Tech A 12:225–232

Taylor RH, Stoianovici D (2003) A survey of medical robotics in computer-integrated surgery. IEEE Trans Robotics Automation 19:765–781

Varkarakis IM, Rais-Bahrami S, Kavoussi LR, Stoianovici D (2005) Robotic surgery and telesurgery in urology. Urology 65(5): 840–846

Chapter 3
Robotic Prostatectomy

Vipul R. Patel, Kenneth J. Palmer, Geoff Coughlin, and Mario F. Chammas

Abstract: In the USA, approximately 77,000 radical prostatectomies are performed yearly for the treatment of prostate cancer. Although a number of alternative treatment options are available for organ-confined prostate cancer, retropubic radical prostatectomy (RRP) remains the gold standard demonstrating a reduction in disease-specific mortality for affected patients.

However, the procedure has inherent morbidity associated with it. Therefore, less invasive surgical techniques have been sought; one such alternative is robotic-assisted laparoscopic radical prostatectomy (RALP). In recent years RALP has become a forerunner in treatment options, yielding comparable medium-term perioperative and functional outcomes.

Robotic-assisted prostatectomy has allowed urologists to enter the realm of minimally invasive surgery by incorporating open-surgery movements to a laparoscopic environment. Current RALP data from several series yield perioperative and functional outcomes comparable to the gold standard. However, long-term data is needed in order to establish its true efficacy.

Using MEDLINE we performed a search for publications on perioperative and functional outcomes related to RALP. We present a review of the available literature.

Keywords: Prostatectomy, Margins, Continence, Potency#

P. Dasgupta (ed.), *Robotic Urological Surgery in Clinical Practice*,   45
DOI: 10.1007/978-1-84800-243-2_3,
© Springer-Verlag London Limited 2008

3.1. Introduction

Cancer of the prostate remains the most common malignancy of the male genitourinary tract. It accounts for nearly 33% of all newly diagnosed cancers in men (Meng et al. 2003). For patients with organ-confined disease a number of treatment alternatives are available. However, RRP remains the gold standard for long-term cure (Myers 2001).

Since its first description in 1905 by H. H. Young this procedure has been associated with significant intraoperative and perioperative morbidity (Young 2002). The technique was revised by Patrick Walsh in the 1980s with an increasing knowledge about the basis of surgical anatomy and has become a refined procedure with acceptable cancer control rates and improved functional outcomes (Reiner and Walsh 1979; Walsh and Lepor 1987). However, it is challenging due to the small confines of the pelvis and its association with higher surgical morbidity caused by the large abdominal incision, postoperative pain, the need for strong narcotic analgesia, and the prolonged recovery period as was reported in a patient complications survey (30% incontinence, 60% erectile dysfunction, and 20% secondary surgical treatments for urethral strictures) (Fowler et al. 1993).

In the minimally invasive surgery era new approaches were being sought after in order to minimize patient morbidity while improving both functional and oncologic outcomes. One viable option was the laparoscopic technique.

The concept of a laparoscopic approach for the treatment of prostate cancer is not new. In the early 1990s Schuessler et al. (Schuessler et al. 1991) described the laparoscopic pelvic lymph node dissection technique. Later, in 1992, Kavoussi and Clayman joined this group to describe their first successful laparoscopic radical prostatectomy (LRP) (Schuessler et al. 1997). Early results were less than promising, with prolonged operative times and no major advantages over conventional surgery (Salomon et al. 2004).

However, the procedure was revived in the late 1990s as European surgeons reevaluated LRP and reported feasibility with results comparable to the open surgical approach (Guillonneau and Vallancien 2000; Rassweiler et al. 2001a; Turk et al. 2001; Eden et al. 2002; Salomon et al. 2002; Rassweiler et al. 2003a). While the technique has become more refined over a 15-year period, it has still failed to become a part of mainstream urology mainly because of its limitations: steep learning curve (minimum of 50–100 cases) and long mean operative times, making it unrealistic for most surgeons. When compared to the open approach, the first series of patients demonstrated no benefit regarding tumor removal, length of hospital stay (LOS), convalescence, continence, potency, or cosmesis (Guillonneau et al. 1999) but since then multiple groups have reported their experiences with outcomes comparable to the former (Guillonneau et al. 2002; Rassweiler et al. 2003b; Trabulsi et al. 2003; Rassweiler et al. 2004).

While the concept of a minimally invasive approach to prostatectomy was attractive, LRP provided certain technical challenges that limited its feasibility, growth and overall rate of adoption. These limitations included two-dimensional vision, counterintuitive motion of the surgeon and non-wristed instrumentation in the confines of the pelvis. It was believed that advances in surgical technology would be necessary to catapult laparoscopy into mainstream urology for prostatectomy. Robotic-assisted surgery has such a potential.

The first robotic prostatectomy was performed in 2000 by Binder in Germany (Binder and Kramer 2001). Subsequently, the procedure has undergone significant innovation and improvement. Menon, Guillonneau, and Vallancien refined the technique at Henry Ford Hospital later in that same year (Pasticier et al. 2001) and its growth has been exponential since then. We present a review of the current state of robotic-assisted laparoscopic prostatectomy (RALP).

3.2. Technique

RALP can be performed via a transperitoneal or preperitoneal technique. The transperitoneal approach is performed by using either a Veress needle or Hasson technique to access the peritoneal cavity. The abdomen is insufflated using CO_2 at 15 mmHg and trocars placed under direct vision, as shown in Fig. 3.1. The patient is then placed in a lithotomy, steep Trendelenburg position and the robot docked (Fig. 3.2).

The procedure is begun using the zero degree binocular lens and the following instruments: monopolar scissors (right arm), PK dissecting forceps (left arm) (Gyrus Group, PLC), and the prograsp (4th arm).

The anterior peritoneum is incised (bladder takedown) to enter the retropubic space of Retzius. The endopelvic fascia is then opened bilaterally and the ani levator fibers peeled off the prostate. Ligation and placement of a suspension stitch with Monocryl 1 on a CT1 needle then follows to stabilize the periurethral complex and aid in early recovery of continence (Fig. 3.3).

Next step in the procedure is the dissection of the bladder neck. This is accomplished by changing the scope to a 30 down angle to improve visualization. Determining the

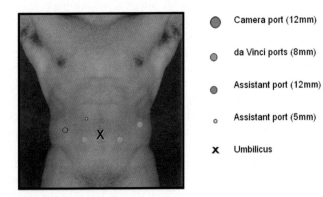

FIGURE 3.1. Port placement.

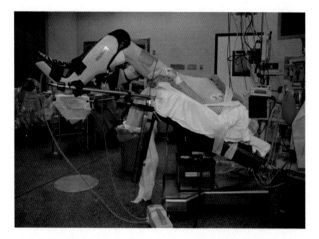

FIGURE 3.2. Lithotomy and steep Trendelenburg position.

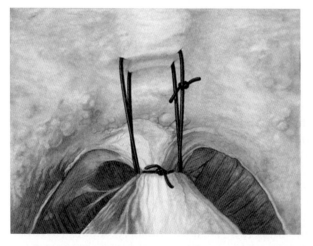

FIGURE 3.3. Ligation and placement of the suspension stitch from the dorsal venous complex to the pubic tubercle. The endopelvic fascia has been opened clearly visualizing the fibers of the levator ani.

boundaries of the prostate and bladder neck can be challenging. A general rule to accomplish this is locating the area where the bladder fat reaches the prostate (no fat on the anterior surface of the prostate). Careful dissection in a downward direction is undertaken until reaching the urethra and catheter. The posterior aspect of the bladder neck is initiated by first retracting the Foley catheter (upward with the 4th arm) and dissecting following the bladder fibers at the precise junction until reaching the vas deferens and seminal vesicles which are transected and dissected, respectively. Denonvillier's fascia is then incised and the posterior rectal plane developed completely leaving the prostate attached only by the pedicles and urethra.

Following the dissection of the posterior plane is the preservation of the neurovascular bundles (NVB) and ligation of the prostate pedicle. These are often a hybrid of various techniques depending on the approach given: antegrade, retrograde, or a combination of the two. Regarding the use of energy during this step, dissection can be athermal or thermal (monopolar, bipolar, harmonics). Another variable factor is the approach to the fascial layers surrounding the prostate at the site of the neurovascular bundle. The approach can be extrafascial, interfascial, intrafascial, or high intrafascial depending on the tumor burden and location.

At our institution, our approach is athermal with an early retrograde release of the NVB that allows precise delineation of the path of the NVB and its relation to the prostate pedicle during ligation of the latter with hemostatic clips reducing the possibility of inadvertent injury during this step (Fig. 3.4).

The apical dissection is then performed using cold scissors to divide the dorsal venous complex (DVC) and urethra. The vesicourethral anastomosis is performed using a modified van Velthoven technique. A single continuous running suture using two 20-cm 3–0 Monocryl sutures (RB1 needle) of different colors are tied together with ten knots. The posterior anastomosis is performed with one arm of the suture beginning at the 5-o'clock position running clockwise to the 10-o'clock position. The anterior anastomosis is completed

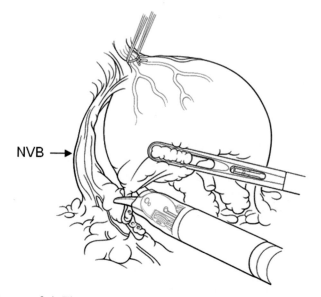

FIGURE 3.4. The path of the neurovascular bundle (NVB) clearly delineated decreasing the possibility of inadvertent injury during ligation of the prostate pedicle with hemostatic clips.

with the second arm of the suture starting in the 5-o'clock position and proceeding in a counterclockwise fashion. Both sutures are tied in the 10-o'clock position on the urethral stump. A Foley catheter is left in place for 4–7 days.

3.3. Outcomes

3.3.1. Operative Time (OR)

A direct comparison between operative times of various series is somewhat difficult due to variations in reporting operative times including setup and/or pelvic lymph node dissection. The mean operative time for reported robotic series ranges from 141–540 min (Abbou et al. 2001; Binder and

Kramer 2001; Pasticier et al. 2001; Rassweiler et al. 2001; Menon et al. 2002a,b; Ahlering et al. 2003; Bentas et al. 2003; Menon and Tewari 2003; Menon et al. 2003; Wolfram et al. 2003; Ahlering et al. 2004; Patel et al. 2005). In our experience, operative time declined from a mean of 202 min for our first 50 cases to141 min for the last 50 in a series of 200 cases (Patel et al. 2005). Analysis of our current data of 1500 consecutive cases shows that OR times have been further reduced to less than 90 min (Palmer et al. 2007). This is also confirmed by Ahlering et al. who reported similar experience-related reduction with a mean of 184 min for their last ten cases compared to an overall of 207 min (Ahlering et al. 2004).

3.3.2. Estimated Blood Loss (EBL) and Transfusion Rate

Traditionally RRP has been associated with higher EBL and transfusion rates. In a comparative study, Menon et al. reported a significantly higher rate of transfusion after RRP (67%) compared to RALP (0%) (Menon et al. 2005a,b). Although diminished blood loss has been the hallmark of laparoscopic prostatectomy, other RALP series have reported mean EBL ranging from 75–900 ml with most being less than 200 ml (Menon and Tewari 2003) and a transfusion rate ranging from 0–16.6% (Abbou et al. 2001; Binder and Kramer 2001; Pasticier et al. 2001; Rassweiler et al. 2001; Menon et al. 2002a,b; Ahlering et al. 2003; Bentas et al. 2003; Menon and Tewari 2003; Menon et al. 2003; Wolfram et al. 2003; Ahlering et al. 2004; Patel et al. 2005).

Several studies have demonstrated that pneumoperitoneum exerts a tamponade effect that aids in diminishing blood loss from venous sinuses. With increasing experience large RALP series like the Vattikuti Institute's and The Ohio State University's report transfusion rates ranging from 0 to 0.4%, respectively (Menon et al. 2007; Palmer et al. 2007).

3.3.3. Length of Hospital Stay

Length of hospital stay is an important component of convalescence after surgery and is often considered a measure of patient well-being. A shorter LOS indicates subjectively a lower degree of morbidity and a faster recovery varying and depending upon the type of surgery, clinical pathway, surgeon practice patterns, and cultural differences. The usual LOS after RRP varies between 1 and 3 days (Kundu et al. 2004). In a single surgeon comparative study, Ahlering et al. reported shorter LOS in patients after RALP compared to RRP (25.9 h vs. 52.8 h) (Ahlering et al. 2004). Similar findings were reported by Tewari et al. with a mean LOS of 1.2 days for the RALP group versus 3.5 days for the RRP group (Tewari et al. 2003). Our current data of 1500 consecutive cases demonstrates a mean LOS of 1.1 days with 97% of the patients being discharged on postoperative day one (Palmer et al. 2007).

3.3.4. Postoperative Pain

As with most minimally invasive procedures, RALP is performed through several small incisions and is associated with minimal postoperative pain. In the few published studies, there are conflicting reports on reduction in postoperative pain with RALP. Menon et al. report that there was a statistically significant difference in visual analog pain score on postoperative day 1 with RALP having a mean score of 3 (1–7) compared to RRP with a mean score of 7 (4–10) (Menon et al. 2007). Webster et al., reported no statistical difference in pain on day of surgery using the Likert pain scale with RALP having a mean score of 2.52 compared to 2.88 in the RRP group (Webster et al. 2005).

3.3.5. Continence

Earlier series of RRP defined incontinence based on patient-reported surveys being as high as 50% (Fowler et al. 1993).

Walsh et al. (Walsh et al. 2000) reported continence (no pad usage in past 4 weeks) to be 54% at 3 months, 80% at 6 months, 93% at 12 months, and 93% at 18 months. The pad free rate after RRP after 3 months of follow-up has been reported to be between 50–76% (Walsh et al. 2000; Lepor et al. 2001; Ahlering et al. 2004).

It has been proposed that RALP can potentially improve continence rates or earlier return of continence by better visualization and preservation of the urethral sphincter and its length. Magnified visualization grants a better and improved preservation of the urethral sphincter allowing the surgeon precise delineation between this structure and the prostatic apex (Smith 2004).

Menon et al. reported a 95.2% continence rate after 12 months following lateral prostatic fascia-sparing RALP in 2652 patients. They also noted that 33% of patients had a >3-point improvement in the IPSS. Continence was defined as "no pads or a single pad for security purposes only and failure to leak urine on provocative maneuvers." At the time of catheter removal 25% of patients were pad free (Menon et al. 2007).

Our initial series of 200 patients was evaluated 2 years ago and we reported continence rates of 47, 82, 89, 92, and 98% at 1, 3, 6, 9, and 12 months, respectively. It was demonstrated that 27% of patients were continent immediately after catheter removal. Continence was defined as "no pads" and the data was collected by an independent third party (Patel et al. 2005).

Ahlering et al. reported on their first 45 RALP cases and subsequently on case numbers 46–105. Sixty-three percent and 81% of patients in their first 45 cases were pad free at 1 and 3 months, respectively. An additional 25% and 14% used a security pad at 1 and 3 months and in the following 60 cases, 76% were pad free at 3 months (Ahlering et al. 2003). Questionnaires were either patient-reported or administered by a nonclinical research associate. In their first 72 RALP cases, Carlsson et al. report that 90% of patients were pad free at 3–6 months postoperatively. Information was gathered by self-administered patient questionnaires (Carlsson et al. 2006).

Analysis of our current series of 1500 cases shows a continence rate of 27, 92, 97, and 97.8% immediately after catheter removal, and at 3, 6, and 12 months, respectively (Palmer et al. 2007). However, in an effort to improve early continence rate we have made several modifications to our technique. The incorporation of a retropubic suspension stitch after ligating the dorsal venous complex we believe stabilizes the periurethral complex and aids in the early recovery of continence. This stitch is passed from right to left between the urethra and DVC, through the periosteum on the pubic bone in a figure-of-eight and then tied (Fig. 3.5). Forty percent of patients who underwent this modification recovered continence in less than 1 month and 92.8, 97.9, and 97.9% at 3, 6, and 12 months, respectively, demonstrating a statistically significant benefit at 3 months ($p = 0.013$). No complications were reported.

Rocco F et al. published data regarding early recovery of continence after RRP by reconstructing the posterior aspect of the rhabdosphincter (Rocco et al. 2007a,b). The technique provides posterior support for the sphincteric mechanism and prevents caudal retraction of the urethra. Continence was defined as the use of no pads or one diaper per day. The early continence rate was 62.4% using this definition. The authors compared the results to a historical group of 50 patients who underwent radical prostatectomy without reconstruction of the rhabdosphincter. The continence rates were significantly better during the first 3 months for the reconstruction group. However, there was little difference following one year. This technique was also applied to LRP by Rocco et al. (Rocco et al. 2007a,b). He performed a prospective trial in which 31 patients had reconstruction while 31 patients had standard laparoscopic prostatectomy. Continence was defined as no pads or the use of one diaper per day. Three days following catheter removal 74.2% of patients in the reconstruction group were continent compared to 25.8% of patients in the standard group. There was a statistically significant better continence rate immediately and 1 month postoperatively.

We have recently incorporated the technique during RALP. Our complete *"early continence"* rate (defined by use

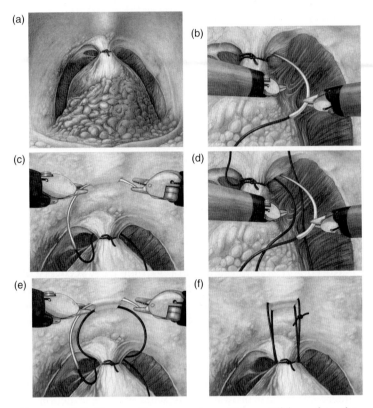

FIGURE 3.5. Retropubic suspension stitch: **a** Vision after the endopelvic fascia has been opened and DVC ligated; **b** CT1 needle held at a 90° angle passed from right to left between the urethra and DVC; **c** stitch placed through the periosteum on the retropubis; **d, e** Second pass through DVC and periosteum; **f** final stitch tied.

of no pads) of 58% at 1 week is encouraging. If the definition of continent is broadened to that of Rocco et al. (0 or 1 pad per day) the rate is 72%. We felt there was a learning curve of approximately 20 cases to perform this modification optimally. During this time we learnt precise identification of the target anatomy and the technical refinements to both the reconstruction and the following urethrovesical anastomosis.

Correct anatomic placement of the distal sutures was the most challenging aspect.

3.3.6. Potency

Theoretically, de novo erectile dysfunction after radical prostatectomy occurs by injury of the neurovascular bundles: thermal or traction, direct incision, or incorporation of the NVBs into hemostatic sutures and/or clips. Several studies have demonstrated that younger age, preoperative potency, comorbidities, and nerve-sparing techniques are key factors affecting the recovery of erectile function (Catalona et al. 1999).

Menon et al. at the Vattikuti Institute in Detroit, recently described and reported potency results for their technique of lateral prostatic fascia-sparing (Veil of Aphrodite) RALP (Menon et al. 2005a,b). These men were evaluated with a self-administered SHIM questionnaire preoperatively and at 12 months postoperatively. Recovery of normal erections was defined as a SHIM score >21. Intercourse was defined by an answer of >2 (sometimes or more often) on question 2 ("when you had erections from sexual stimulation, how often were your erections hard enough for penetration?"). Using these criteria, 70 and 100% of men with a preoperative SHIM score >21 reported normal erections and intercourse at 12 and 48 months, respectively. Fifty percent of them attained normal SHIM score without medication.

Chien et al. reported early sexual outcomes using a clipless nerve-sparing RALP technique. Sexual outcomes were evaluated with the use of a self-reported validated questionnaire preoperatively and at 1, 3, 6, and 12 months postoperatively. While 80 patients underwent RALP during this study period, 35 patients were excluded from final analysis due to either follow-up <3 months, open conversion, or incomplete questionnaires. It was found that after 1 month postoperatively the patient's sexual function scores had returned to 47% of their preoperative scores. This increased to 54, 66, and 69% at 3, 6, and 12 months postoperatively. Also reported was a subjective sexual potency, defined as "the ability to penetrate and complete intercourse with or without the use of oral PDE-5 inhibitors." Using this definition, 50% (ten men) of patients undergoing bilateral nerve sparing RALP were potent and 44% (eight men) of patients undergoing unilateral bilateral nerve sparing RALP were potent (at 6 months follow-up) (Chien et al. 2005).

After a 9-month follow-up of their first 45 RALPs, Ahlering et al. reported that one out of three patients who were preoperatively potent had satisfactory postoperative sexual function with sildenafil (Ahlering et al. 2003). Using a cautery-free neurovascular bundle dissection, they also reported early potency outcomes. A comparison was made between patients undergoing unilateral or bilateral nerve preservation (23/45) and 36 "controls" (standard bipolar cautery dissection). Erectile function was assessed through self-administered questionnaires and defined as erections sufficient for vaginal penetration with or without PDE-5 inhibitors. After 3 months of follow-up, 43% of men in the cautery-free group were potent compared with 8.3% of the control group. While longer follow-up for the cautery-free group is awaited, the authors commented that at 16 months follow-up 60% of the control group were potent (Ahlering et al. 2005).

At our institution the approach to prostatectomy is antegrade in the standard manner. However, we have modified our nerve-sparing technique in order to provide the least trauma to the neurovascular bundle. Our approach to the nerve sparing is athermal with early retrograde release of the NVB, interfascial or intrafascial depending upon tumor burden and location (Fig. 3.6).

Between March 2006 and December 2006, 332 patients with localized prostate cancer underwent nerve-sparing RALP by the modified technique (Palmer et al. 2007). A bilateral nerve-sparing procedure was performed in 201 (60.5%) patients, unilateral nerve sparing in 60 (18.2%)

(a)
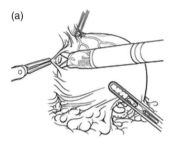

(b)
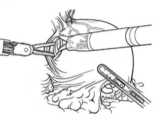

(c)
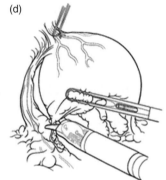

(d)
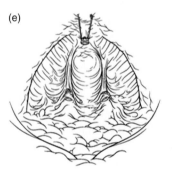

(e)

FIGURE 3.6. Neurovascular bundle (NVB) preservation. **a** A first incision is made in the mid-lateral aspect of the prostatic fascia; **b** Dissection plane is encountered with minimal bleeding from small tributary vessels; **c** Ligation of the prostate pedicle with hemostatic clips; **d** NVB has been completely dissected and prostate pedicle clipped and transected; **e** Bilateral NVB preservation after removal of the prostate specimen.

and non-nerve sparing in 71 (21.3%) patients. Out of these patients, 167 patients with preoperative SHIM score >17, who underwent a unilateral or bilateral nerve-sparing procedure and had at least 3 months of postoperative follow-up, were included in the review. Out of 167 patients, 134 (80%) patients were potent with or without use of PDE 5 inhibitors. Fifteen (9%) patients were potent immediately after catheter removal, 46 (27.5%) were potent at 1-month follow-up, 115 (68.8%) were potent at 3-months follow-up, 133 (79.6%) were potent at 6-months follow-up, and 134 (80%) were potent after 12 months of follow-up.

In their first 100 RALP, Mikhail et al. report obtaining 68% and 79% of potency in patients who underwent unilateral or bilateral nerve preservation, respectively, after a 12-month follow-up excluding those with preoperative impotence, sural nerve grafting, or those with nonsparing procedures (Mikhail et al. 2006).

Some authors have conducted single institute comparisons between RALP and either RRP or LRP. Tewari et al. reported a prospective comparison between 100 RRPs and 200 RALPs demonstrating a more rapid return of erections with RALP (50% at a mean follow-up of 180 days vs. 50% at a mean of 440 days after RRP) as well as a quicker return to intercourse with RALP (50% at 340 days vs. 50% at 700 days for RRP). While this study has many strong points, the authors do acknowledge that one team performed the RALPs while eight different surgeons performed the RRPs (Tewari et al. 2003). Joseph et al. retrospectively compared 50 LRPs and 50 RALPs. While their data was immature 22% of the LRP patients reported erections compared to 40% in the RALP group (Joseph et al. 2005).

3.3.7. Oncologic Outcomes

The reported positive margin rates (PMR) after RALP series range from 0–36%. When stratified by stage, PMRs following RALP range from 0–17% for T2a,

0–33% for T2b, 0–82% for T3a, 20–50% for T3b, and 33–67% for T4 (Guillonneau et al. 2002). Although no statistical significance was demonstrated, Ahlering et al. reported a trend toward a higher rate of PMRs in the RRP group (20%) compared to the RALP group (16.7%) (Ahlering et al. 2004).

In our first series of 200 patients the PMR for T2, T3a, T3b, and T4 tumors was 5.7, 29, 20, and 33%, respectively (Patel et al. 2005). As our technique was refined and after the current 1500 consecutive cases we have seen a reduction in our PMRs: 4% for pT2, 34% for T3, and 40% for pathologic stage T4. The distribution of positive surgical margins was: apex (23%), bladder neck (14.5%), posterolateral (36.7%), and multifocal (26%). When analyzing the rate of positive margins based on final pathologic prostate volume, we found that in patients with prostate volumes of less than 50 g, 50–99 g, and greater than or equal to 100 g, positive margin rates were 14.3, 9.4, and 5.9%, respectively.

For RALP to be accepted as a satisfactory alternative to the current gold standard, oncologic outcomes must be proven to be uncompromised.

3.3.8. Safety

Experience has shown that patients often seem concerned about the safety of using the robot. We conducted a multi-institutional study in which experienced surgeons reported failures of the da Vinci™ surgical system. Data collected comprised a total case volume of 6426 and median surgeon experience of 460 cases (325–1500). Critical failures of the system that led to canceling ten cases and conversion to one laparoscopic and nine open procedures occurred in 20 cases (0.3%; range 0–1.1%) and recoverable failures occurred in 124 cases (2.2%). The most common sites of system malfunction were the optical system and surgical arms. Although technical problems can occur, this study demonstrates that robotic equipment malfunction is extremely rare in institutions that perform high volumes of RALPs (Lavery et al. 2007).

There are currently over 600 robotic systems in the United States and over 30,000 robotic procedures have been performed (personal communication with Intuitive Surgical, Inc. VRP). Twenty-five percent of all prostatectomies were performed robotically in 2005 and it is estimated that about 60% will be performed this way in 2007.

Our review represents a comprehensive analysis of our data and of that of other series available in the surgical literature. Perioperative and functional outcomes provided by larger series for robotic radical prostatectomy are encouraging. In addition, there appears to be a trend toward earlier return of function in those undergoing robotic surgery. While this is encouraging we acknowledge that the data is short term and longer follow-up is needed in these patients. As techniques continue to evolve and an increasing number of larger series are published, we anticipate that the results of robotic radical prostatectomy will continue to improve.

3.4. Conclusions

Robotic-assisted laparoscopic radical prostatectomy is a procedure in evolution. Our review of the literature suggests that it is associated with shorter OR time, decreased blood loss and transfusion rate, shorter LOS, less pain and promising continence, potency and oncologic outcomes when compared to contemporary RRP and LRP series. Although robotics is still in its infancy and there are no long-term follow-up studies, many international series have demonstrated that there appears to be an earlier return of continence and recovery of potency in patients undergoing this type of surgery. More information will be available as series continue to mature. With continued refinement of the operative technique we will see further improvement in outcomes.

References

Abbou CC, Hoznek A et al. (2001) Laparoscopic radical prostatectomy with a remote controlled robot. J Urol 165(6 Pt 1): 1964–1966

Ahlering TE, Skarecky D et al. (2003) Successful transfer of open surgical skills to a laparoscopic environment using a robotic interface: initial experience with laparoscopic radical prostatectomy. J Urol 170(5):1738–1741

Ahlering TE, Woo D et al. (2004) Robot-assisted versus open radical prostatectomy: a comparison of one surgeon's outcomes. Urology 63(5):819–822

Ahlering TE, Eichel L et al. (2005) Rapid communication: early potency outcomes with cautery-free neurovascular bundle preservation with robotic laparoscopic radical prostatectomy. J Endourol 19(6):715–718

Bentas W, Wolfram M et al. (2003) Robotic technology and the translation of open radical prostatectomy to laparoscopy: the early Frankfurt experience with robotic radical prostatectomy and one year follow-up. Eur Urol 44(2):175–181

Binder J, Kramer W (2001) Robotically-assisted laparoscopic radical prostatectomy. BJU Int 87(4):408–410

Carlsson S, Nilsson A et al. (2006) Postoperative urinary continence after robot-assisted laparoscopic radical prostatectomy. Scand J Urol Nephrol 40(2):103–107

Catalona WJ, Carvalhal GF et al. (1999) Potency, continence and complication rates in 1,870 consecutive radical retropubic prostatectomies. J Urol 162(2):433–438

Chien GW, Mikhail AA et al. (2005) Modified clipless antegrade nerve preservation in robotic-assisted laparoscopic radical prostatectomy with validated sexual function evaluation. Urology 66(2):419–423

Eden CG, Cahill D et al. (2002) Laparoscopic radical prostatectomy: the initial UK series. BJU Int 90(9):876–882

Fowler FJ, Jr., Barry MJ et al. (1993) Patient-reported complications and follow-up treatment after radical prostatectomy. The National Medicare Experience: 1988–1990 (updated June 1993). Urology 42(6):622–629

Guillonneau B, Cathelineau X et al. (1999) Laparoscopic radical prostatectomy: technical and early oncological assessment of 40 operations. Eur Urol 36(1):14–20

Guillonneau B, Vallancien G (2000) Laparoscopic radical prostatectomy: the Montsouris experience. J Urol 163(2): 418–422

Guillonneau B, Cathelineau X et al. (2002) Laparoscopic radical prostatectomy: assessment after 550 procedures. Crit Rev Oncol Hematol 43(2):123–133

Joseph JV, Vicente I et al. (2005) Robot-assisted vs pure laparoscopic radical prostatectomy: are there any differences? BJU Int 96(1):39–42

Kundu SD, Roehl KA et al. (2004. Potency, continence and complications in 3,477 consecutive radical retropubic prostatectomies. J Urol 172(6 Pt 1):2227–2231

Lavery HJ, Thaly RK et al. (2007) Robotic equipment malfunction during robotic prostatectomy: A multi-institutional study. Urology 70(Suppl. 3A)

Lepor H, Nieder AM et al. (2001) Intra-operative and postoperative complications of radical retropubic prostatectomy in a consecutive series of 1,000 cases. J Urol 166(5):1729–1733

Meng MV, Elkin EP et al. (2003) Predictors of treatment after initial surveillance in men with prostate cancer: results from CaPSURE. J Urol 170(6 Pt 1):2279–2283

Menon M, Shrivastava A et al. (2002a) Laparoscopic and robot assisted radical prostatectomy: establishment of a structured program and preliminary analysis of outcomes. J Urol 168(3): 945–949

Menon M, Tewari A et al. (2002b) Prospective comparison of radical retropubic prostatectomy and robot-assisted anatomic prostatectomy: the Vattikuti Urology Institute experience. Urology 60(5):864–868

Menon M, Tewari A (2003a) Robotic radical prostatectomy and the Vattikuti Urology Institute technique: an interim analysis of results and technical points. Urology 61(4 Suppl 1):15–20

Menon M, Tewari A et al. (2003b) Vattikuti Institute prostatectomy: technique. J Urol 169(6):2289–2292

Menon M, Kaul S et al. (2005a) Potency following robotic radical prostatectomy: a questionnaire based analysis of outcomes after conventional nerve sparing and prostatic fascia sparing techniques. J Urol 174(6):2291–2296, discussion 2296

Menon M, Shrivastava A et al. (2005b) Laparoscopic radical prostatectomy: conventional and robotic. Urology 66(5 Suppl): 101–104

Menon M, Shrivastava A et al. (2007) Vattikuti Institute prostatectomy: contemporary technique and analysis of results. Eur Urol 51(3):648–657; discussion 657–658

Mikhail AA, Stockton BR et al. (2006) Robotic-assisted laparoscopic prostatectomy in overweight and obese patients. Urology 67(4):774–779

Myers RP (2001) Radical prostatectomy: making it a better operation in the new millennium. Int J Urol 8(7):9–14

Palmer KJ, Shah K et al. (2007) Robotic assisted laparoscopic radical prostatectomy: Peri-operative outcomes of 1500 consecutive cases. Urology 70(Suppl. 3A):136

Pasticier G, Rietbergen JB et al. (2001) Robotically assisted laparoscopic radical prostatectomy: feasibility study in men. Eur Urol 40(1):70–74

Patel VR, Tully AS et al. (2005) Robotic radical prostatectomy in the community setting—the learning curve and beyond: initial 200 cases. J Urol 174(1):269–272

Rassweiler J, Frede T et al. (2001a) Telesurgical laparoscopic radical prostatectomy. Initial experience. Eur Urol 40(1):75–83

Rassweiler J, Sentker L et al. (2001b) Heilbronn laparoscopic radical prostatectomy. Technique and results after 100 cases. Eur Urol 40(1):54–64

Rassweiler J, Seemann O et al. (2003a) Technical evolution of laparoscopic radical prostatectomy after 450 cases. J Endourol 17(3):143–154

Rassweiler J, Seemann O et al. (2003b) Laparoscopic versus open radical prostatectomy: a comparative study at a single institution. J Urol 169(5):1689–1693

Rassweiler J, Schulze M et al. (2004) Laparoscopic radical prostatectomy: functional and oncological outcomes. Curr Opin Urol 14(2):75–82

Reiner WG, Walsh PC (1979) An anatomical approach to the surgical management of the dorsal vein and Santorini's plexus during radical retropubic surgery. J Urol 121(2):198–200

Rocco B, Gregori A et al. (2007a) Posterior reconstruction of the rhabdosphincter allows a rapid recovery of continence after transperitoneal videolaparoscopic radical prostatectomy. Eur Urol 51(4):996–1003

Rocco F, Carmignani L et al. (2007b) Early continence recovery after open radical prostatectomy with restoration of the posterior aspect of the rhabdosphincter. Eur Urol 52(2):376–383

Salomon L, Levrel O et al. (2002) Radical prostatectomy by the retropubic, perineal and laparoscopic approach: 12 years of experience in one center. Eur Urol 42(2):104–110; discussion 110–111

Salomon L, Sebe P et al. (2004) Open versus laparoscopic radical prostatectomy: part I. BJU Int 94(2):238–243

Schuessler WW, Vancaillie TG et al. (1991) Transperitoneal endosurgical lymphadenectomy in patients with localized prostate cancer. J Urol 145(5):988–991

Schuessler WW, Schulam PG et al. (1997) Laparoscopic radical prostatectomy: initial short-term experience. Urology 50(6): 854–857

Smith JA, Jr. (2004) Robotically assisted laparoscopic prostatectomy: an assessment of its contemporary role in the surgical management of localized prostate cancer. Am J Surg 188(4A Suppl):63–67

Tewari A, Srivasatava A et al. (2003) A prospective comparison of radical retropubic and robot-assisted prostatectomy: experience in one institution. BJU Int 92(3):205–210

Trabulsi EJ, Hassen WA et al. (2003) Laparoscopic radical prostatectomy: a review of techniques and results worldwide. Minerva Urol Nefrol 55(4):239–250

Turk I, Deger IS et al. (2001) Laparoscopic radical prostatectomy. Experiences with 145 interventions. Urologe A 40(3):199–206

Walsh PC, Lepor H (1987) The role of radical prostatectomy in the management of prostatic cancer. Cancer 60(3 Suppl): 526–537

Walsh PC, Marschke P et al. (2000) Patient-reported urinary continence and sexual function after anatomic radical prostatectomy. Urology 55(1):58–61

Webster TM, Herrell SD et al. (2005) Robotic assisted laparoscopic radical prostatectomy versus retropubic radical prostatectomy: a prospective assessment of postoperative pain. J Urol 174(3):912–914; discussion 914

Wolfram M, Brautigam R et al. (2003) Robotic-assisted laparoscopic radical prostatectomy: the Frankfurt technique. World J Urol 21(3):128–132

Young HH (2002) The early diagnosis and radical cure of carcinoma of the prostate. Being a study of 40 cases and presentation of a radical operation which was carried out in four cases. 1905. J Urol 168(3):914–921

Chapter 4
Comparison of Robotic Laparoscopic and Open Radical Prostatectomy

Evangelos Liatsikos, Panagiotis Kallidonis, Jens-Uwe Stolzenburg, Roger Kirby, and Christopher Anderson

Abstract: Over the years radical prostatectomy has evolved from open to laparoscopic to robotic-assisted. This chapter provides a critical review and comparison of all three techniques. Non-randomised outcomes appear to support lower positive margin rates and better erectile function with robotic surgery. These results, however, are as much dependent on surgical expertise as on technological advances.

Keywords: Radical prostatectomy, Retropubic, Laparoscopic, Robotic, Margins, Continence, Potency

4.1. Introduction

Prostate cancer is the most common malignant disease and the second leading cause of cancer death (Dijkman and Debruyne 1996; Parker et al. 1996). The introduction of the anatomic basis of nerve-sparing open retropubic radical prostatectomy (RRP) by Walsh and Donker in 1982 rendered the surgical treatment of localized prostate cancer effective and acceptable (Walsh and Donker 1982). Through the years, the experience gained contributed to the modification and

P. Dasgupta (ed.), *Urologic Robotic Surgery in Clinical Practice*,
DOI: 10.1007/978-1-84800-243-2_4,
© Springer-Verlag London Limited 2008

refinement of the initial technique. Nevertheless, the main principles remained the same (Walsh et al. 1983; Catalona 1985; Walsh 1998; Kirby et al. 2006).

The first laparoscopic radical prostatectomy (LRP) using a transperitoneal approach was performed by Schuessler et al. in 1992 with disappointing results in terms of operative time (Schuessler et al. 1992). The experience gained with the new technique forced the latter group to conclude in 1997 that LRP did not offer any advantage in comparison with the RRP (Schuessler et al. 1997). Raboy et al. introduced the extraperitoneal approach for LRP and Gaston et al. also initiated performing LRP in the same year (1997) (Raboy et al. 1997). However, the first promising experience with LRP was reported by Guillonneau et al. in 1998 and triggered worldwide interest in minimal invasive surgery (Guillonneau et al. 1999; Guillonneau and Vallancien 2000). Several European centers followed the steps of the above pioneers (Jacob et al. 2000; Bollens et al. 2001; Rassweiler et al. 2001b; Stolzenburg et al. 2002). In course of time, technical improvements refined and standardized LRP resulting in diminished morbidity (Rassweiler et al. 2003; Stolzenburg et al. 2003; Salomon et al. 2004).

In the USA, the urologic community confronted LRP with skepticism. The acceptance of the technique by the American centers was very limited (Raboy et al. 1997; Gill and Zippe 2001). The cooperation of the pioneering team of Guilloneau and Vallancien with Menon contributed to the expansion of LRP in the USA (Menon et al. 2002).

Laparoscopic digital imaging provides advantages in visualization of the operative field such as magnification and illumination. Nevertheless, important disadvantages exist. Excellent hand-to-eye coordination is necessary in order for the surgeon to overcome the paradoxical movement of the instruments, tactile feedback is very limited, the images are two dimensional, and the surgeon should adapt to the new anatomic perspectives. As a result, LRP is accompanied by a long learning curve, requiring more than 40 procedures to be mastered under a well-organized training program (Blanna et al. 2007; Stolzenburg et al. 2006a). The above facts led to the idea of the application of robots in an effort to improve the precision and accuracy of the anatomic dissection.

Binder and Kramer performed the first robotic-assisted laparoscopic radical prostatectomy (RALP) in 2000 (Binder and Kramer 2001). Successful RALP was also performed by Pesticier et al. in the Vattikuti Institute soon after (Pasticier et al. 2001). The technique was further developed in the following years by the same group (Menon et al. 2002). The introduction of the da Vinci^{TM} robotic surgical system® (Intuitive Surgical, Inc., Sunnyvale, California) allowed nonlaparoscopic surgeons to perform a laparoscopic prostatectomy (Smith 2004). When a RALP is performed by an experienced open surgeon, the learning curve appears to be accelerated. Similar results have been reported by both academic (Menon et al. 2003a) and community settings (Patel et al. 2005). Robotic assistance enabled both laparoscopically experienced and naïve surgeons to accomplish a RALP in comparable time with LRP within 10 to 20 cases (Menon et al. 2003b; Ahlering et al. 2004b; Patel et al. 2005). The above facts contributed to the acceptance of the RALP in the USA and led the urologic interest towards minimally invasive prostatectomy.

The robotic system provides a combination of the excellent visualization capabilities of digital laparoscopes with the additional advantage of three-dimensional imaging and the Endowrist^{TM} technology which is responsible for the increased freedom of movement of the instruments. In fact, the rigidity of the instrument shaft and the fixed position of the trocar (Fig. 4.1) on the abdominal wall limit the freedom of movement to four in the case of LRP. The Endowrist^{TM} provides articulated instruments which allow six degrees-of-freedom (Matsunaga et al. 2006). Tremor control and motion scaling is also an advantage of the system by allowing the surgeon to customize the function of the robotic system. On the contrary, a major disadvantage remains the complete absence of tactile feedback (Matsunaga et al. 2006).

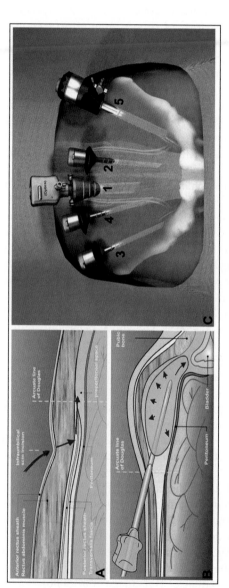

FIGURE 4.1. Dissection of the preperitoneal space and Trocar placement for extraperitoneal laparoscopic approach. **A** Landmarks for the dissection of the preperitoneal space. The space between the rectus muscle and the posterior rectus sheath is first of all bluntly developed by finger dissection. **B** Balloon trocar insertion and insufflation creating the retroperitoneal working space under direct visual control. **C** Sequence of placement of trocars .Notice the course of the epigastric vessels on both sides.

4.2. Technical Aspects

Retropubic radical prostatectomy is based on the initial technique proposed by Walsh and Donker with minor modification varying from center to center and two nerve-sparing techniques, the antegrade and retrograde approach (Goad and Scardino 1994; Montorsi et al. 2005; Graefen 2006; Barre 2007).

On the other hand, during LRP or RALP techniques the removal of the prostate gland can be performed in an ascending (from the apex to the base) or descending fashion (from base to apex). An issue of technical debate is the approach to use to perform the operation. Some centers favor the transperitoneal approach (e.g, Institut Mutualist Montsouris, France; Klinikum Heilbronn, Germany; Vattikuti Institute, USA; University of California at Irvine, USA), other urologic groups prefer the extraperitoneal access (Erasme Hospital, Belgium; Leipzig University, Germany). It should be noted that most of the large series of RALP reported, have been performed according to the intraperitoneal descending method described by the Montsouris Group with modifications (Tewari et al. 2002; Perer et al. 2004). Experience with the extraperitoneal approach is currently limited (Antiphon et al. 2003; Dakwar et al. 2003; Gettman et al. 2003).

The extraperitoneal descending technique is considered to have a shorter learning curve which is presented by shorter operative time (Bollens et al. 2005; Poulakis et al. 2005; Rassweiler et al. 2006b). The main advantages of the approach are the lower risk of bleeding due to control of the lateral prostatic pedicles (Fig. 4.2) in an early stage of the descending procedure and the absence of the initial retrovesical dissection of the seminal vesicles in the extraperitoneal versus transperitoneal descending technique. The elimination of the latter step is responsible for 50 min reduction of the operative time as reported by Hoznek et al. (Hoznek et al. 2001). The balloon dissection of the space of Retzius also reduces operative time. Nevertheless, all other steps of the prostatectomy procedure are

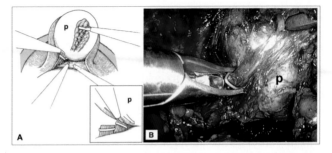

FIGURE 4.2. Prostatic pedicle dissection for extraperitoneal approach. During dissection of left prostatic pedicle, the assistant retracts the partially mobilized prostate to the right side (**A**), and vice versa. The prostatic pedicle and small vessels are clipped and divided between Endoclips (**B**). Care has to be taken to avoid inadvertent injury to the neurovascular bundle. It is advisable to proceed with the clipping and cutting in small steps (*inlay*). p = prostate.

performed independent of the approach used and it would be expected that the operative time in experienced hands is similar (Rassweiler et al. 2006a). Management of patient characteristics and technical problems may be more favorable with one approach than the other. For instance, a history of extensive pelvic surgery or redundant sigmoid colon represents a difficult case for the transperitoneal ascending technique in order to expose the pouch of Douglas. Likewise, the early division of the dorsal vein complex with the ascending technique is probably more difficult in the case of patients with large prostates (Rassweiler et al. 2006a). Comparable results between extraperitoneal and transperitoneal approaches have been reported, but there is no consensus among the investigators on the ideal approach (Catalona and Smith 1998; Han et al. 2001; Salomon et al. 2002; Menon et al. 2003a; Roumeguere et al. 2003; Cathelineau et al. 2004b). Hoznek et al. and Ruiz et al. propose that the extraperitoneal approach is more favorable due to the reduced bowel injury, ileus, and peritonitis (Hoznek et al. 2003; Ruiz et al. 2004). On the other hand, Erdogru et al. and Cathelineau et al. report

TABLE 4.1. Comparison studies between extraperitoneal and transperitoneal LRP

Author	Number	Operative time (min)	Complications (%)	Transfusion (%)	Reintervention (%)	Catheter time (days)	Positive margins
Hoznek et al. 2001	40						
–Transperitoneal	20	224	Non Available	15	5	5.3	15
–Extraperitoneal	20	170	7.3	10	—	4.2	25
Cathelinaeu 2003	200						
–Transperitoneal	100	173	23.8	4	—	6.2	26.2
–Extraperitoneal	100	163	16.7	3	—	6	15.9
Ruiz et al. 2004	330						
–Transperitoneal	165	248	Non Available	1.2	Non Available	5.1	23
–Extraperitoneal	165	220	Non Available	5.4	Non Available	6.6	Non Available
Erdogru 2004	106						
–Transperitoneal	53	187	24.6	13	1.8	7	20.7
–Extraperitoneal	53	191	11.8	16	—	7	22.6
Brown et al. 2005	156						
–Transperitoneal	122	197	10.7	3	Non Available	Non Available	24
–Extraperitoneal	34	191	11.8	—	Non Available	Non Available	21
Remzi et al. 2005	80						
–Transperitoneal	39	279	20	Non Available	7.7	Non Available	25.6
–Extraperitoneal	41	217	37	Non Available	2.4	Non Available	19.5

that no significant differences between the two techniques exist and the whole issue is a "false debate" (Cathelineau et al. 2004a; Endogru et al. 2004). The literature data are summarized in Table 4.1

Certain advantages characterize each of the procedures. The transperitoneal access is related to larger space of the operative field, less tension on the vesicourethral anastomosis, and minimal risk to lymphocele formation, especially in the case of extended pelvic lymph node dissection. The extraperitoneal approach avoids any contact with the bowel, thus time-consuming lysis of adhesions is avoided and the risk of bowel injury is diminished. Moreover, urine extravasation tends to be less problematic in case of extraperitoneal approach due to the fact that the extravasated urine is not within the peritoneal cavity. An extraperitoneal approach in patients with gross obesity has the advantage of shorter distance between trocar insertion site and operative field. Considering the above, the parallel approach of both techniques in centers of expertise in LRP has been proposed by Rassweiler et al. (2006a).

Despite the different techniques performed, the main goal of radical prostatectomy remains the excision of cancer with the least morbidity and the maximum potential for a full recovery of continence and potency, important functional factors for the quality of life (QoL) of the operated patients. Every technique is evaluated under the light of the above requirements (Rassweiler et al. 2006a).

4.3. Perioperative Results

4.3.1. Operative Time

One of the main points of criticism against LRP and RALP is the longer operative time accompanying both procedures compared to open surgery (Omar and Townell 2004). All comparative studies between LRP and RRP reveal longer operative time for the former technique. The operative time ranges were 180–330 min for LRP and 105–197 min for RRP.

The reports comparing LRP and RRP perioperative data are summarized in Table 4.2. Frede et al. (2005) observed a decrease of operative time from 332 min to 196 min when comparing the first cases with the last 50 cases, thus it could be proposed that the operative time is related to the experience of the surgeon performing the operation, a fact that is also observed during laparoscopic training schemes (Stolzenburg et al. 2006a). Nevertheless, the introduction of the extraperitoneal approach was accompanied by a decrease of operative time resulting in the reproduction of operative time similar to those of RRP (Stolzenburg et al. 2003; Anghel et al. 2005; Poulakis et al. 2005). Mean operative time for RALP as presented by El-Hakim and Tewari after the summary of the existing data on RALP was 222 min (El-Hakim and Tewari 2004). The experience of Patel et al. gained from a series of 200 consecutive patients in a community setting revealed mean operative time of 141.2 min (Patel et al. 2005). Menon et al. reported a mean operative time of 160 min accompanied by excellent continence and potency outcome. Similar results have not been reproduced by any other group (Rassweiler et al. 2001a; Bentas et al. 2003; Wolfram et al. 2003; Cathelineau et al. 2004b).

4.3.2. Complications and Morbidity

LRP is accompanied by lower blood loss in comparison with RRP (Table 4.3). All comparative studies concur with the latter observation with the exception of one. The average estimated blood loss ranged between 189 ml and 1100 ml for LRP, while RRP blood loss was 550–1550 ml. Blood transfusion rate was also lower in the case of LRP (Rassweiler et al. 2006a). The Montsouris group reported a mean blood loss of 380 ml and an allogeneic transfusion in 4.9% of cases while there was no autologous blood transfusion for the 550 patients operated with LRP (Guillonneau et al. 2002a). Eden et al. reported an estimated blood loss rate of 313 ml and allogeneic transfusion rate of 3% (Eden et al. 2002). The highest blood loss was observed in the Rassweiler et al. series with

TABLE 4.2. Comparative studies of laparoscopic versus retropubic radical prostatectomy

Author	Number of patients	Operative time (min)	Complications (%)	Reintervention (%)	Analgesics (mg)	Blood loss (ml)	Transfusion (%)
Guilloneau 2001	220						
−RRP	100	135	Non available	Non available	Non available	850	31
−LRP	120	239	7.3	2.5	Non available	402	10
Salomon et al. 2002	401						
−RRP	219	197	23.8	Non available	Non available	Non available	26.2
−LRP	219	285	18.1	Non available	Piritramid	Non available	2.9
Rassweiler et al. 2003	657						
−RRP	219	196	19.1	6.8	50.8	1550	55.7
−LRP early	219	288	13.9	4.2	33.8	1100	30.1
−LRP late	219	218	6.1	2	30.1	800	9.6
Roumeguere et al. 2003	162						
−RRP	77	168	24.6	7.8	Non available	1514	Non available
−eLRP	85	288	11.8	3.5	Non available	522	Non available
Artibani et al. 2003	121						

TABLE 4.2. Continued

Author	Number of patients	Operative time (min)	Complications (%)	Reintervention (%)	Analgesics (mg)	Blood loss (ml)	Transfusion (%)
–RRP	50	105	20	4	Non available	Non available	34
–LRP	71	180	37	4.2	Non available	Non available	63
Brown et al. 2005	120						
–RRP	60	Non available	18.3	3.3	Non available	1355	52
–LRP	60	330	25	3.3	Non available Tramadol	317	1.7
Remzi et al. 2005	121						
–RRP	41	195	Non available	7.3	300	385	Non available
–LRP	39	279	Non available	7.7	290	290	Non available
–eLRP	41	217	Non available	2.4	189	189	Non available

TABLE 4.3. Summary of complication data between RRP and LRP (Rassweiler et al. 2003, 2006a)

Complication	RRP	LRP
Transfusion rate	0.3–1.4	0.3–8.9
Rectal lesion	0.2–2.3	1.5–2.5
Ureter lesion	0.3–0.5	0–0.3
Dehiscent anastomosis	0.2–0.4	0–0.2
Lymphocele	1.7–2.9	0–2.2
Disturbed wound healing	0.9–3.4	0.2–0.7
Thromboembolic incidents	0.6–1.9	0.6–1.5

an average volume of 430 ml and a transfusion rate of 30% for the first 219 cases. The respective figures for the last cases were 800 ml and 9.6% (Rassweiler et al. 2003). It should be noted that the authors attributed the high blood loss to the ascending technique during which the dorsal vascular complex dissection and ligation as well as the transaction of the urethra are performed early. On the contrary, both steps are performed last in the retrograde approach (Guillonneau et al. 1999). According to El-Hakim and Tewari's summary of the existing data on RALP, the average estimated blood loss was 231 ml and the blood transfusion rate 0.3% (El-Hakim and Tewari 2004). Patel et al. reported that estimated blood loss in their series was 75 ml and no transfusion was required (Patel et al. 2005).

A lower incidence of complications with LRP in comparison to RRP has been demonstrated by Frede et al. and Rassweiler et al. (Rassweiler et al. 2004, 2006b; Frede et al. 2005). Complications like bleeding, urine extravasation, wound healing, and thromboembolic incidents are summarized in Table 4.3. A comparison of the data presented in two large series with an identical number of patients ($n = 1243$) confirmed the lower complication rate of LRP over RRP (Table 4.4). After the performance of 567 consecutive LRPs

TABLE 4.4. Comparison of the incidence of different complications after open and laparoscopic radical prostatectomy in large series

Complication	RRP (1243 patients)	LRP (1243 patients)
	University of Hamburg, Augustin et al. 2002 (%)	Heilbronn Clinic, Rassweiler et al. 2006a (%)
Major Complications	10.7	12.3
–Intraoperative	6.6	8.9
–Transfusion rate	6.1	7.7
–Rectal lesion	0.2	1.2
–Ureter lesion	0.3	–
–Postoperative	4.1	3.6
–Cardiovascular	0.6	0.1
–Thromboembolic	1.3	0.3
–Infections	0.5	–
–Lymphocele	0.6	–
–Renal	0.2	0.9
Minor Complications	15.8	3.4
–Nervous System	1.1	0.3
–Thromboembolic	0.3	0.1
–Gastrointestinal	0.4	0.2
–Pulmonary system	0.6	0.1
–Renal	0.6	0.2
–Lymphocele	2.3	–
–Urine retention	1.7	1
–Wound dehiscence	1.4	0.1
–Prolonged lymph drainage	1.3	0.3
–Pelvic hematoma	0.7	0.5
–Cardiovascular	1.1	–

at Montsouris over a period of 3 years, the total complication rate was 17%, with 4% and 14.6% of major and minor complications, respectively. Major complications requiring reintervention were bowel and rectal injury in 1% of the cases, hemorrhage in 1%, and ureteral injuries in 0.3% of cases (Geary et al. 1995). Gonzalgo et al. designed a grading system for the detailed report of frequency and severity of complications following LRP (Gonzalgo et al. 2005). In a population of 246 patients undergoing LRP, 34 morbidities were observed (13.8%). Most of the incidents were self-limiting (94.1%) and categorized as grade II and III according to the system applied. Only 5.9% (n = 2) were grade IV which represents potential life-threatening events requiring intensive care unit management. Grade V complications (death) did not occur. Conversion and reintervention rates were less than 1%. El-Hakim and Tewari revealed a minor complication rate of 4.55% in RALP including urinary tract infection, anastomotic leaks, ileus, and port site bleeding. Major complications took place in 3.75% including deep vein thrombosis, pulmonary emboli, obturator nerve injury, anastomotic disruption, delayed bleeding, and wound dehiscence (El-Hakim and Tewari 2004). Patel et al. in a community setting reported a 2% complication rate with two cases of rectal injuries, a case of hematoma, and a bladder neck contracture (Patel et al. 2005).

Probably, the most severe complication of radical prostatectomy is rectal injury. The incidence ranges between 1 and 2% of LRP and occurs often during the apical dissection during a wide excision of the prostate. It is important to recognize any rectal injury intraoperatively because adequate repair solves the problem without consequences. An overseen rectal injury can result in fistulae and peritonitis, making temporary colostomy essential (Rassweiler et al. 2001c, 2003).

4.3.3. Conversion to Open Surgery

In a multi-institutional study reporting 1228 cases, Sulser et al. reported low conversion rates in all major series reflecting the careful introduction of LRP (Sulser et al. 2001). The experience gained is helpful in overcoming challenging situations like managing cases following previous laparoscopic hernioplasty (Endogru et al. 2005). Furthermore, technical reasons such as adhesions, difficulty with the urethrovesical anastomosis, and malfunctioning of instruments as well as risk of positive surgical margins due to uncertain tumor anatomy are the causes of open conversion rather than intraoperative complications (bleeding, visceral injury) (Rassweiler et al. 2006b). Bhayani et al. reported a 1.9% conversion rate in a multi-institutional series and noted prior pelvic surgery and morbid obesity as contributing factors (Bhayani et al. 2004). In RALP series, the conversion rate is about 1% (El-Hakim and Tewari 2004), while the experience gained by a large community series showed no requirement for open conversion (Patel et al. 2005).

4.4. Comparison of Oncologic Results

4.4.1. Surgical Margin

Radical prostatectomy aims at the complete surgical removal of the entire prostate, its surrounding fascia, and the seminal vesicles. Pelvic lymphadenectomy accompanies the prostatectomy procedure when indicated (Scardino 2005). The presence of cancer at the inked margin of resection on the prostatectomy specimen is defined as a positive surgical margin (PSM) (Wieder and Soloway 1998). The positive predictive value of frozen section analysis for positive surgical margins is high. However, the sensitivity is too limited considering the fact that a routine frozen section analysis of the suspicious sites is unable to reduce PSM rates significantly (Tsuboi et al. 2005). The prognostic value of a PSM is reflected by a higher risk of biochemical recurrence, local and systemic progression (Catalona and Smith 1998; Cathelineau et al. 2004b). Factors influencing PSMs include the preoperative serum PSA (prostate-specific antigen) level, Gleason grade, clinical stage, the surgeon and surgical technique as well as patient selection (Ruiz et al. 2004; Brown et al. 2005).

Reports on pathologic and oncologic results are presented in Table 4.5. The Montsouris group reported the experience gained with the first 1000 LRP cases achieving an overall PSM rate of 19.2%. The respective rates for pT2, pT3 disease were 15.5 and 31% (Guillonneau et al. 2003). The experience of the Heilbronn group with 500 cases reported an overall PSM rate of 19%, 7.4% for pT2, and 31.8% for pT3 disease (Rassweiler et al. 2005b). The Charitè group after performing 1000 LRPs observed PSM rates of 14.8 and 54.4% for pT2 and pT3 tumors, respectively (Lein et al. 2006). The University of Leipzig reported PSMs in 9.8% of the pT2 tumor specimens and 34.4% of the pT3 in a series of 1300 consecutive extraperitoneal endoscopic radical prostatectomies (Stolzenburg et al. 2007). The above results reflect the experience of high-volume centers including the first cases when the LRP technique was under development and the surgeons inexperienced in the new procedure.

Large series of patients who underwent RALP are few and limited to certain centers. Moreover, the presented data on the RALP often differ from the standards of preceding series of LRP. The Vattikuti Institute reported the results on 2652 cases of RALP achieving an overall PSM of 13% (Menon et al. 2007). Columbus University observed PSM rates of 9.9% for pT2 and 32.7% for pT3 tumors after 325 procedures (Joseph et al. 2006). Ahlering et al. reported average PSM rates of 5.2% for pT2 and 37.6% for pT3 tumors (Ahlering et al. 2006). Patel et al. (2006) in a study of 500 RALP cases reported an overall PSM rate of 9.4%. The PSM rates were 2% for T2a, 4% for T2b, 2.5% for T2c, 23% for T3a, 46% for T3b, and 53% for T4. Organ-confined tumor specimens were detected to have PSMs in 2.5% of the cases and nonorgan confined specimens 31%.

An interesting issue was the high incidence of PSM rates during the initial cases with both LRP and RALP (Rassweiler et al. 2001b; Ahlering et al. 2004a; Atug et al. 2006).

TABLE 4.5. Open vs. Laparoscopic vs. Robotic radical prostatectomy oncologic results

Authors (year)	N of patients	Positive margins			PSA recurrence 0.2 ng/ml				Clinical progress	
					3 years		5 years			
		pT2	Total	pT3	pT2	pT3	pT2	pT3	After 3 years	After 5 years
Open radical prostatectomy										
Catalona	1,778		20.9		7.5	21.3	10.0	31.3	NA	4.5
Han	2,494	NA		26.4	15.0	25.0	25.0	40.0	NA	4.0
Hull	1,000		12.8		4.4	14.7	5.1	24.7	NA	10.1
Salomon	264	16.4		44.3	6.8	42.0	NA	NA	NA	NA
Roumeguere	77	7.3		67.7	6.9[a]	14.7[a]	NA	NA	NA	NA
Harris	508	2.1		47.8	3.7[b]	33.1[b]	NA	NA	6.9	NA
Touijer	692	5.3		22.0	NA	NA	NA	NA	NA	NA
Chun	2708		11 / 21.5		8.5	41.1	11.5	55.9	NA	NA
Laparoscopic radical prostatectomy										
Salomon	137	21.9		40.8	9.6	43.2	NA	NA	NA	NA
Roumeguere	85	7.8		45.7	8.6[a]	11.4[a]	NA	NA	NA	NA]
Guillonneau	1,000	15.5		31.1	11.0	33.0	NA	NA	NA	NA]
Rassweiler	500	7.4		31.8	4.1	12.0[c]	NA	NA	2.0	NA
Rassweiler	500	7.4		31.8	4.8	28.5	10.5	31.9 (+pT4)	4.1	9.8
Lein	938	14.8		54.4	5.2	21.4 (+pT4)	NA	NA	NA	NA
Stolzenburg	491	10.8		31.2	NA	NA	NA	NA	NA	NA
Goemann et al.	550	17.9		44.8	9	NA	10.3	41.4	NA	NA
German Study Group, Rassweiler	3,535	10.6 [3.2–18.0]		pT3a 32.7 [20.0–38.5] pT3b 56.2 [40.0–75.0]	8.6 [4–15.3]	17.5 [15 20.6]	NA	NA	NA	NA

TABLE 4.5. Continued

Authors (year)	N of patients	Positive margins			PSA recurrence 0.2 ng/ml				Clinical progress	
		pT2	Total	pT3	3 years		5 years		After 3 years	After 5 years
					pT2	pT3	pT2	pT3		
Toutijer	485	8.2		17.2	NA	NA	NA	NA	NA	NA
Rozet	599	14.6		25.6	5[a]	NA	NA	NA	NA	NA
Stolzenburg	1,187 conv	9.8		34.3	NA	NA	NA	NA	NA	NA
	113 intra	6.1		20.0						
Robotic-assisted radical prostatectomy (RALP)										
Wolfram	81	12.7		42.0	NA	NA	NA	NA	NA	NA
Menon	100	10.6		40.0	NA	NA	NA	NA	NA	NA
Tewari	200		6.0 [pT2a–pT3a]		8.0[d]		NA	NA	NA	NA
Menon	565		23.0	48.8	NA	NA	NA	NA	NA	NA
Ahlering	140	12.3			11.4[f]		NA	NA	NA	NA
	Cases 1–50	27.3		50.0						
	Cases 51–140	4.7		44.0						
Patel	200	9.9		32.7	6[e]		NA	NA	NA	NA
Joseph	325	9.9		32.7	2.3[g]		NA	NA	NA	NA
Atug	140	18.1		54	NA		NA	NA	NA	NA
	Cases 1–33	38.4		60						
	Cases 34–66	13.7		66						
	Cases 67–140	3.6		40						
Atug	40 TP	9.6		44.4	NA		NA	NA	NA	NA
	40 EP	10.3		45.5						
Esposito	625		17		5[h]		NA	NA	NA	NA
Ahlering	1,090	5.2 [2.4–8.5]		37.6 (25.5–46.3)	NA	NA	NA	NA	NA	NA

TABLE 4.5. Continued

Authors (year)	N of patients	Positive margins			PSA recurrence 0.2 ng/ml				Clinical progress	
					3 years		5 years			
		pT2	Total	pT3	pT2	pT3	pT2	pT3	After 3 years	After 5 years
Slawin	ORP 504	3.1		13.6	NA	NA	NA	NA	NA	NA
	RALP127	6.2		22	NA	NA	NA	NA	NA	NA
Zorn	300	15.1		52.1	3.2[i]	26.1[i]	NA	NA	NA	NA
Samadi	70	18		36	7[j]		NA	NA	NA	NA
		1.5			Gleason 6	1.5		Gleason 6 1.5		
Menon	2,652				Gleason 7	4.6	2.3	Gleason 7 4.6	NA	NA
					8 and 9	8.2	overall	8 and 9 39.9		

NA not available, conv conventional, intra intrafascial
[a] Results at 1 year
[b] 4 years
[c] 24% of pT3 with adjuvant therapy
[d] Results at 9 months
[e] At 9.7 months (median)
[f] 3 months
[g] 6 months
[h] 2 years
[i] 17.8 months (median)
[j] 7 months (median)

Nevertheless, the accumulation of surgical experience contributed to the decrease of surgical margin rates for both techniques (Ahlering et al. 2006; Atug et al. 2006; Menon et al. 2007). The latter phenomenon was also observed during the development of the open radical prostatectomy. Overall, a PSM rate of 10% seems to be highly acceptable. Moreover, no definitive advantage for one surgical approach over the other in terms of PSM rates was noted when the existing data on different methods and surgical experience were compared (Table 4.5). Surgical experience seems to be the most important factor for the PSM rates as was noted in the German Laparoscopic Working Group after the evaluation of 5824 cases. The technique performed was not related to the pathologic outcome of the procedure (Galli et al. 2006). An effort to overcome the long learning curve and to improve oncologic and functional results through the establishment of mentoring programs is reflected in the numerous articles published (Patel et al. 2005; Ahlering et al. 2006; Joseph et al. 2006; Rassweiler et al. 2006b; Touijer et al. 2006; Menon et al. 2007; Stolzenburg et al. 2007).

4.4.2. PSA Recurrence

PSA recurrence is a marker used to evaluate cancer control. Definition of PSA values related to tumor progression is variable between the authors and the PSA value representing tumor recurrence ranges from 0.1 to 0.4 ng/ml (Wieder and Soloway 1998; Guilloneau 2006; Stolzenburg et al. 2007). Short-term PSA recurrence data accompanying the LRP and RALP techniques are similar to those reported in the RRP literature. However, long-term cancer control data are unavailable.

Biochemical recurrence free rates in LRP series after 3-years follow-up were noted to be 90.5% as reported by Guilloneau et al. (PSA level <0.1 ng/ml). The respective figures for pT2a, pT2b, pT3a, and pT3b were 91.8, 88, 77, and 44%, respectively. In the case of nodal metastases, the disease free rate as represented by the biochemical recurrence of PSA was 50% (Guillonneau et al. 2003). Rassweiller et al. observed an overall freedom from biochemical progression rate of 83% at 3 years and 73.1% at 5 years (two PSA values >0.2 ng/ml) (Rassweiler et al. 2005b).

Long-term oncologic results are not available for patients that underwent RALP. Short-term data are similar to those of RRP and LRP (Table 4.5). In general, the oncologic outcome of the recently developed techniques seems to be similar. Nevertheless, long-term follow-up data are necessary in order for the scientific community to be convinced for the above issue.

In general, surgical margin remains as an independent predictor of biochemical recurrence in a multivariate setting. Nevertheless, the predictive value is low. PSMs do not necessarily represent the existence of cancer in the operated site and moreover do not drive the prognosis alone. In fact, early organ-confined tumors have excellent prognosis regardless of PSM status. On the contrary, advanced cancers such as seminal vesicle involvement have bad prognosis regardless of the surgical margin status. Margin status is independently related to the outcome when taken into account with Gleason grade, capsular penetration, and seminal vesicle involvement. An independent association with margin status does not exist in cases of total or high-grade cancer volumes (Graefen 2006).

4.5. Comparison of Functional Results

The lack of uniformity in defining, assessing, and reporting functional results following radical prostate excision is responsible for the inability to compare existing series objectively. Differences in the definition of parameters, methodology of data collection and evaluation time leads to confusion in data interpretation and generally in disparity between the reported results.

4.5.1. Continence

Guilloneau et al. and Stolzenburg et al. used the validated International Continence Society questionnaire for the data collection and interpretation of continence in their LRP series. The report of Guilloneau et al. in 2002 on a series of 550 patients with 12-months follow-up revealed that 82.3% of the patients were pad free, 12% needed one pad a day, and 5.9% had urinary incontinence requiring more than two pads a day (Guillonneau et al. 2002a). Stolzenburg et al. in a series of 1300 extraperitoneal LRPs after 12-months follow-up observed 91.9% to be pad free, 6.9% needing one pad a day, and 1.2% requiring more than two pads a day (Stolzenburg et al. 2007). Table 4.6 shows the existing literature on continence results after the performance of RRP, LRP, and RALP.

Stanford et al. investigated the recovery of continence in 1291 patients after 24-month follow-up in the Prostate Cancer Outcomes Study (PCOS). Total urinary control was reported in 31% of the patients while 60.5% were pad free and 14.3% considered their urinary incontinence to be a moderate to big problem (Stanford et al. 2000). It is obvious that patient questionnaires reveal far worse results than the surgeons' database (Begg et al. 2002; Bianco et al. 2005). RALP series introducing continence terms like "social dryness" and "security liner" represent an obstacle in the effort to compare results (Menon et al. 2007). Some authors propose that both laparoscopic and robotic laparoscopic approaches as methods to perform radical prostatectomy are probably not responsible for any differences in continence rates. Nevertheless, surgical experience along with technical refinements may lead to better continence results (Eastham et al. 1996). Technical modifications such as bladder neck or puboprostatic as well as intrapelvic branch of the pudendal nerve preservation, reconstruction of the rectourethralis muscle or structures of the rectourethral fascia are still under question. The issue of early continence has been raised, but remains in doubt due to the bias of the total continence reported (Table 4.7) (Rassweiler et al. 2004; Takenaka et al. 2006).

TABLE 4.6. Reported recovery of continence rates following ORP, LRP, and RALP

Reference	Total patients	Mean age (years)	Method of assessment	Definition used (pads)	Time of assessment (months)	Continence rate (%)
Open radical prostatectomy (ORP)						
Leandri	620	68.0	P	0–1	12	95.0
Geary	456	64.1	P	0	>18	80.1
Eastham	390	51–75	P	0–1	24	95.0
Davidson	170	63.0	Q	0–1	12	85.9
Feneley	177	63.0	P	0–1	12	97.0
Talcott	94	61.5	Q	0	12	61.0
Bates	83	65.0	Q	0	22	76.0
Catalona	1,325	63.0	P	0–1	50	92.0
Kleinhans	44	68.0	P	0	12	97.7
Steiner	593	34–76	P	0	12	94.5
Walsh	64	57.0	Q	0	18	93.0
Stanford	1,291	62.9	Q	tc	12	31.0
				0	12	61.0
Kao	1,069	63.6	Q	0	>12	77.0
Sullivan	75	63.3	Q	0	12	87.0
Rassweiler	219	65.0	Q	0	12	89.9
Roumeguere	77	63.9	P	0	12	83.9
Artibani	50	64.3	P	0	12	78.5
Harris	439	65.8	P	0	12	96.0
Laparoscopic radical prostatectomy (LRP)						
Hoznek	200	64.8	Q	0	12	86.0

TABLE 4.6. Continued

Reference	Total patients	Mean age (years)	Method of assessment	Definition used (pads)	Time of assessment (months)	Continence rate (%)
Türk	275	60.2	P	0–1	12	94.0
Salomon	100	65.1	Q	0	12	90.0
Eden	100	62.2	P	0	12	90.0
Guillonneau	550	63.0	Q	0	12	82.0
Anastasiadis	230	64.1	Q	0	12	71.6
Roumeguere	85	62.5	Q	0	12	80.7
Stolzenburg	70	63.4	P	0	6	90.0
Artibani	50	64.3	P	0	12	60.0
Rassweiler	310	64.0	Q	0	24	97.7
Rozet	600	NA	Q	0	12	84.0
Stolzenburg	700	63.4	Q	0	12	92.0
German Study Group, Rassweiler	5,824	64.0	Q	0	12	84.9 [72–94]
Goemann	550	62.4	Q	0	12	82.9
Galli	150	64.0	Q	0	12	91.7
Lein	952	62.0	Q	0–1	28	76.0
	1,205 std				3	67.9
	1,140 std				6	85.0
Stolzenburg	995 std	63.4	Q	0	12	91.9
	intra 49				12	91.8

TABLE 4.6. Continued

Reference	Total patients	Mean age (years)	Method of assessment	Definition used (pads)	Time of assessment (months)	Continence rate (%)
Robotic-assisted radical prostatectomy (RALP)						
Menon	100	60.0	P	0–1	6	92.0
Tewari	200	59.9	Q	0	12	91.0
Ahlering	60	62.9	Q	0	1w	33.0
					1	63.0
					3	81.0
Menon	565	NA	Q	0	6	96.0
Patel	200	59.5	Q	0	12	98.0
					1w	28.0
Joseph	325	60.0	NA	0	3	93.0
					6	96.0
Esposito	625	56.1	Q	0	12	86.0
Zorn	300	59.2	Q	0	12	90.2
Menon	2,652	60.2	NA	0–1	12	95.2
Samadi	70	60.3	Q	0	3	76.0

P Physician, Q Questionnaire, w week, intra intrafascial, std standard, NA no data available, tc total control

TABLE 4.7. Regaining of continence after radical prostatectomy over time in ORP, LRP, and RALP

Follow-up	ORP		LRP			RALP	
	Eastham	Harris	Salomon	Stolzenburg	Rassweiler	Menon	Joseph
1 month (%)	28	38	45	NA	28	50[a]	28
3 months (%)	65	62	63	67.9	51	90[a]	93
6 months (%)	79	85	74	85	70	NA	96
12 months (%)	92	96	90	91.9	84	95.2[a]	NA
24 months (%)	95	NA	NA	NA	97	NA	NA

In other words, the available data on continence after RRP, LRP, and RALP are difficult to compare and all suffer from the same bias. Considering the complexity of the issue investigated, it is at least expected that the urologic community establishes a unified methodology and terminology for the field (Guilloneau 2006).

4.5.2. Erectile Function

Preservation of the erectile function after the performance of a radical prostatectomy is based on the precise and adequate separation of the cavernous nerves in the neurovascular bundle (Fig. 4.3) from the prostate (Walsh and Donker

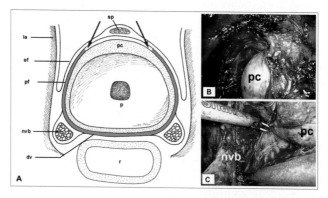

FIGURE 4.3. Intrafascial preservation of the neurovascular bundles for extraperitoneal approach. Schematic depiction of cross section through prostate to give anatomic relations of prostate, endopelvic fascia, periprostatic fascia, Denonvilliers' fascia, and neurovascular bundles (**A**). Dissection plane for intrafascial nerve sparing is shown in *blue* (*arrows*). The "shining" surface of the prostatic capsule is clearly seen laterally (**B**) as well as posteriorly (**C**). The periprostatic fascia and the neurovascular bundle can be separated from the prostatic capsula by blunt dissection in most cases. p = prostate, la = levator ani muscle, nvb = neurovascular bundles, sp = Santorini plexus, pc = prostatic capsule, ef = endopelvic fascia, pf = periprostatic fascia, dv = Denonvilliers' fascia, r = rectum.

1982). The understanding of the anatomic course of the above nerves is important in the effort to preserve potency. Principles of the anatomic dissection are independent of the surgical approach. Nerve-sparing techniques were developed after the understanding of the anatomic structures (Kaul et al. 2005; Graefen et al. 2006; Kirby et al. 2006; Stolzenburg et al. 2006b; Takenaka et al. 2006, 2007; Tewari et al. 2006). The existing techniques preserve the neurovascular bundles during the excision. However, the introduction of the intrafascial and "veil of Aphrodite" technical modifications aim to preserve more neural tissue and to improve the functional outcome. The contribution of the recent refinements to potency preservation remains questionable (Rassweiler 2006). The role of laparoscopic magnification or precision of surgical instruments for the performance of a more accurate and less traumatic dissection of the neurovascular bundles and consequently the achievement of better potency results remains unclear. Unfortunately, the comparison of the erectile function results is also difficult due to the absence of uniformity in the methods used for collection and interpretation of data (Salomon et al. 2004; Rozet et al. 2006).

Differences in the terms defining potency, such as the ability to achieve spontaneous erections or the successful performance of intercourse, are responsible for the difficulty in comparing existing studies. Moreover, the population size, patient characteristics, and multiple factors affecting potency (e.g., medical comorbidities, available sexual partner) as well as the use of additional therapies (PDE-5 inhibitors or vasoactive injections) influence the potency rates of the studies and contribute to the above problem (Briganti and Montorsi 2006). It should be noted that the short-term potency rates are not representative of the final result, thus the recovery to sexual function after a nerve-sparing radical prostatectomy requires up to 48 months and the current data should be discussed with care (Rabbani et al. 2004).

Numerous studies on the field of erectile function after radical prostatectomy have been performed and are presented in Table 4.8 (Guillonneau et al. 2002a; Su et al. 2004;

TABLE 4.8. Recovery of potency after bilateral preservation in ORP, LRP, and RALP

Authors (year)	Total N	Eval Pat. N	Mean age (years)	Percentage of patients receiving BNS	Time of assessment	Potency (%)
Open radical prostatectomy						
Talcott	94	19	61.5	42.4	12	48.0
Catalona	1,870	798	63.0	86.1	18	21.0
Stanford	1,291	1,042	62.9	NA	18	68.0
Walsh	64	64	57.0	100	18	44.0
Roumeguere	77	51	63.9	42.9	12	86.0
						54.5
Graefen	1,755	542	NA	NA		90.0
						56.0
Laparoscopic radical prostatectomy						
Hoznek	200	82	64.8	32.0	1	46.0
Türk	125	44	59.9	11.0	12	59.0
Salomon	235	43	63.8	39.5	12	58.8
Eden	100	100	62.2	58.0	12	62.0
Guillonneau	550	47	NA	NA	1.5	66.0
Anastasiadis	230	230	64.1	33.5	12	53.0
Stolzenburg	70	40	63.4	7.5	2	66.7
Roumeguere	85	85	62.5	30.9	12	65.3
Su	177	173	57.8	51.4	12	48.0
Rassweiler	500	109	67.0	37.6	12	67.0

TABLE 4.8. Continued

Authors (year)	Total N	Eval Pat. N	Mean age (years)	Percentage of patients receiving BNS	Time of assessment	Potency (%)	
Rozet	600	231	NA	60.2	6	64.0	
Stolzenburg	700	185	63.4	10.1	6	47.0	
Wagner	220	220	58.0	66	12	72.0	
German Study Group	5,824	NA	64.0	NA	12	52.5	
Rassweiler						>60	56
						<60	78.8
Goemann	550	NA	62.4	67.0	12	>60	60.6
					24	<60	90.0
Stolzenburg	1,300	367	63.4	17.6	12	69.0	
Robotic-assisted laparoscopic prostatectomy							
Menon	250	200	59.9	NA	6	64.0	
Tewari	200	NA	59.9	100	12	84.0	
						<60 yrs 64.0	
Menon	565	NA	NA	100	6	>60 yrs 38.0	
Joseph	325	150	60.0	86.0	6	68.0	

TABLE 4.8. Continued

Authors (year)	Total N	Eval Pat. N	Mean age (years)	Percentage of patients receiving BNS	Time of assessment	Potency (%)
Esposito	625	160	56.1	NA	24	70.0
					12	58.0
					48	62.0
Menon	2,652	1,142	60.2	Stand. 42.0	12	70.0
				Veil 33.0	48	100
					1	36.0
Zorn	300	161	59.4	62.0	6	61.0
					12	80.0

NA not available
[a]Uni– and bilateral nerve sparring
[b]Without PDG5, veil "veil of Aphrodite"
[c]IIEF-5 score of 22–25

Menon et al. 2007). As a general advice avoidance of hemostatic energy sources (e.g., electrocautery) and the performance of meticulous interfascial dissection with preservation of the cavernous nerves are recommended. The aforementioned technical refinements play a critical role in the optimal postoperative recovery of erectile function (Ong et al. 2004; Su et al. 2004; Rassweiler et al. 2006b).

4.6. Quality of Life

Quality of life after RRP has been well investigated but remains poorly documented (Hara et al. 2003; Link et al. 2005; Rassweiler et al. 2005a; Söderdahl et al. 2005). Söderdahl et al. (2005) observed that 70.7 versus 71% of the patients who underwent LRP and RRP, respectively, returned to baseline urinary function 12 months after the operation. The respective figures for return to baseline erectile function were 42.9 and 39%. The same group also reported no significant difference between non- or nerve-sparing (unilateral or bilateral) neurovascular bundle preservation. Link et al. revealed an average recovery rate to baseline urinary and sexual function of 67 and 64%, respectively (Link et al. 2005). QoL improved in 7.8% and remained stable in 37.4% of the first 500 patients who underwent LRP by the Heilbronn group (Hara et al. 2003). Salomon et al. introduced a score to analyze the global results of radical prostatectomy (Salomon et al. 2003). The absence of biochemical progression (0–4), incontinence (0–2), and impotence (0–1) were taken into consideration. The score one year after radical prostatectomy was 7 for 20% of the patients, 6 for 35.1% of them. These data were based on PSA below 0.2 ng/ml in 85%, continence in 65.8%, and erections in 32.7% of the patients. The application of the Salomon score by Rassweiler et al. in 217 patients who underwent LRP revealed similar figures (score 7 = 22.1%, score 6 = 47.9%). The latter group proposed the extension of the Salomon scoring system to include postoperative complications and a realistic baseline for each patient depending on individual tumor stage, age, and postoperative erectile function (Rassweiler et al. 2005a).

4.7. Economic Considerations

Equipment expenses and longer operative time are responsible for the higher operating room cost of minimally invasive prostatectomy in comparison to RRP (Lotan et al. 2004; Link et al. 2005). Robotic-assisted surgery is clearly the most expensive approach. The latest equipment costs approximately 1.5 million Euros and the yearly maintenance is about 150,000 Euros. The multiple use but disposable robotic instruments cost 600–1000 Euros per case. Lotan et al. estimated a lower cost of $487 and $1726 for RRP in comparison with LRP and RALP, respectively (Lotan et al. 2004). Menon et al. proposed in 2005 that an institution must perform at least 75 cases per year with an average operative time of 3 hours per case in order for the application of the robotic system to be cost effective (Menon et al. 2003b).

Link et al. estimated the factors influencing the overall costs. The most important was the length of hospital stay and the second most important the consumable items such as laparoscopic equipment and trocars (Link et al. 2005). Cost equivalence has already been reached between LRP and RRP due to the use of reusable items (Rozet et al. 2006; Menon et al. 2007). The operative time for LRP has been reduced to 2.5 hours similar to the duration of open surgery (Poulakis et al. 2005; Stolzenburg et al. 2007). The increased cost of the minimally invasive procedures is offset by the shorter hospital stay in comparison to the open approach (Patel et al. 2005; Burgess et al. 2006; Menon et al. 2007).

4.8. Conclusions

Considering the above results on oncologic and functional outcome as well as the lower morbidity of LRP and RALP, it seems certain that the urologic interest will move gradually towards the minimally invasive techniques. Surgeons favoring the above methods are awaiting the long-term results in order to overcome the criticisms on the oncologic potential of the techniques. Robotic surgery is probably the way of the future due to the combination of the excellent characteristics of laparoscopy and the ability to perform with precision, accuracy, and increased dexterity. The superior visualization is also an advantage. The major obstacle to be overcome remains the high cost.

References

Ahlering TE, Skarecky D, Lee D, Clayman RV (2003) Successful transfer of open surgical skills to a laparoscopic environment using a robotic interface: initial experience with laparoscopic radical prostatectomy. J Urol 170(5):1738–1741

Ahlering TE, Eichel L, Edwards RA, Lee DI, Skarecky DW (2004a) Robotic radical prostatectomy: a technique to reduce pT2 positive margins. Urology 64(6):1224–1228

Ahlering TE, Woo D, Eichel L, Lee D, Edwards R, Skaresky D (2004b) Robot-assisted versus open prostatectomy: a comparison of one surgeon's outcomes. Urology 64:819–822

Ahlering TE, Patel V, Columbus OH, David IL, Philadelphia PA, Douglas S, Orange CA (2006) Multi-Institutional Review of Pathological Margins after Robot-Assisted Laparoscopic Prostatectomy (RLP). AUA abstract [1158]

Anastasiadis AG, Salomon L, Katz R, Hoznek A, Chopin D, Abbou CC (2003) Radical retropubic versus laparoscopic prostatectomy: a prospective comparison of functional outcome. Urology 62(2):292–297

Anghel G, Maldonado R, Safi K, Erdogru T, Teber D, Frede T, et al. (2005) Laparoscopic radical prostatectomy—comparison of the operative time of different generations of surgeons. Eur Urol Suppl4(3):244 [Abstract 968]

Antiphon P, Hoznek A, Gettman M, la Taille A, Solomon L, Katz R, Borkowski T, Abbou C (2003) Extraperitoneal laparoscopic robot assisted radical prostatectomy. J Urol 169 [Abstract V965]

Artibani W, Grosso G, Novara G, Pecoraro G, Sidoti O, Sarti A, Ficarra V (2003) Is laparoscopic radical prostatectomy better than traditional retropubic radical prostatectomy? An analysis of peri-operative morbidity in two contemporary series in Italy. Eur Urol 44(4):401–406

Atug F, Castle EP, Srivastav SK, Burgess SV, Thomas R, Davis R (2006) Positive surgical margins in robotic-assisted radical prostatectomy: impact of learning curve on oncologic outcomes. Eur Urol 49(5):866–871

Augustin H, Hammerer P, Graefen M, Palisar J, Noldus J, Fernandez S, et al. (2002) Intraoperative and perioperative morbidity of contemporary radical retropubic prostatectomy in consecutive series of 1243 patients: results of a single center between 1999 and 2002. Eur Urol 43:113–118

Barre C (2007) Open radical retropubic prostatectomy. Eur Urol 52:71–80

Bates TS, Wright MP, Gillatt DA (1998) Prevalence and impact of incontinence and impotence following total prostatectomy assessed anonymously by the ICS-male questionnaire. Eur Urol 33(2):165–169

Bianco FJ Jr, Riedel ER, Begg CB, Kattan MW, Scardino PT (2005) Variations among high volume surgeons in the rate of complications after radical prostatectomy: further evidence that technique matters. J Urol 173(6):2099–2103

Binder J, Kramer W (2001) Robotically-assisted laparoscopic radical prostatectomy. BJU Int 87(4):408–410

Begg CB, Riedel ER, Bach PB, Kattan MW, Schrag D, Warren JL, Scardino PT (2002) Variations in morbidity after radical prostatectomy. N Engl J Med 346(15):1138–1144

Bentas W, Wolfram M, Jones J, Brautigam R, Kramer W, Binder J (2003) Robotic technology abd the translation of open radical prostatectomy to laparoscopy: The early Frankfurt experience with the robotic radical prostatectomy and one year follow up. Eur Urol 44:175–181

Bhayani SB, Pavlovich CP, Strup SE, Dahl DM, Landman J, Fabrizio MD, et al. (2004) Laparoscopic radical prostatectomy: a multi-institutional study of conversion to open surgery. Urology 63:99–102

Blanna A, Straub M, Wild PJ, Lunz JC, Bach T, Wieland WF, Ganzer R (2007) Approach to endoscopic extraperitoneal radical prostatectomy (EERPE): the impact of previous laparoscopic experience on the learning curve. BMC Urol 7:11

Bollens R, Vanden Bossche M, Rhoumeguere Th, Damoun A, Ekane S, Hoffmann P, Zlotta AR, Schulman CC (2001) Extraperitoneal laparoscopic radical prostatectomy: results after 50 cases. Eur Urol 40:65–69 12

Bollens R, Sandhu S, Roumeguere T, Quackels T, Sculman C (2005) Laparoscopic radical prostatectomy: the learning curve. Curr Opin Urol 15:1–4

Briganti A, Montorsi F (2006) Penile rehabilitation after radical prostatectomy. Nat Clin Pract Urol 3(8):400–401 88

Brown JA, Robin D, Lee B, Dahl DM (2005) Transperitoneal versus extraperitoneal approach to laparoscopic radical prostatectomy: an assessment of 156 cases. Urology 65:320–324

Burgess SV, Atug F, Castle EP, Davis R, Thomas R (2006) Cost analysis of radical retropubic, perineal, and robotic prostatectomy. J Endourol 20(10):827–830

Catalona WJ (1985) Nerve-sparing radical retropubic prostatectomy. Urol Clin North Am 12(1):187–199

Catalona WJ, Smith DS (1998) Cancer recurrence and survival rates after anatomic radical retropubic prostatectomy for prostate cancer: intermediate-term results. J Urol 160:2428–2434

Catalona WJ, Carvalhal GF, Mager DE, Smith DS (1999) Potency, continence and complication rates in 1,870 consecutive radical retropubic prostatectomies. J Urol 162:433–438

Cathelineau X, Cahill D, Widmer H, Rozet F, Baumert H, Vallacien G (2004a) Transperitoneal or extraperitoneal approach for laparoscopic radical prostatectomy: a false debate over a real challenge. J Urol 171:714–716

Cathelineau X, Rozet F, Vallancien G (2004b) Robotic radical prostatectomy: the European experience. Urol Clin North Am 31:639–699

Chun FK, Graefen M, Zacharias M, Haese A, Steuber T, Schlomm T, Walz J, Karakiewicz PI, Huland H (2006) Anatomic radical retropubic prostatectomy-long-term recurrence-free survival rates for localized prostate cancer. World J Urol 24(3):273–280

Dakwar G, Ahmed M, Sawczuk I, Rosen J, Lanteri V, Esposito M (2003) Extraperitoneal robotic prostatectomy: comparison of technique and results at one institution. J Urol 169: [Abstr 1660]

Davidson PJ, van den Ouden D, Schroeder FH (1996) Radical prostatectomy: prospective assessment of mortality and morbidity. Eur Urol 29(2):168–173

Dijkman GA,Debruyne FM (1996) Epidemiology of prostate cancer. Eur Urol 30:281–295

Eastham JA, Kattan MW, Rogers E, Goad JR, Ohori M, Boone TB, Scardino PT (1996) Risk factors for urinary incontinence after radical prostatectomy. J Urol 156(5):1707–1713

Eden CG, Cahill D, Vass JA, Adams TH, Dauleh MI (2002) Laparoscopic radical prostatectomy: the initial UK series. BJU Int 90(9):876–882

El-Hakim A and Tewari A (2004) Robotic prostatectomy- a review. MedGenMed (online) 6(4):20

Endogru T, Teber D, Frede T, Marrero R, Hammady A, Seemann O, et al. (2004) Comparison of transperitoneal and extraperitoneal laparoscopic radical prostatectomy using match pair analysis. Eur Urol 46:312–20

Endogru T, Teber D, Frede T, Marrero R, Hammady A, Rassweiler J (2005) The effect of previous transperitoneal laparoscopic herniorrhaphy on trans peritoneal laparoscopic radical prostatectomy. J Urol 173:769–772

Esposito M, Ahmed M, Dakwar G, Lanteri V (2006) Pure extraperitoneal laparoscopic robotic prostatectomy (EP-LRP): a large series experience. AUA abstract [1148]

Feneley MR, Gillatt DA, Hehir M, Kirby RS (1996) A review of radical prostatectomy from three centres in the UK: clinical presentation and outcome. Br J Urol 78(6):911–8; 919–20

Frede T, Erdogru T, Zulosky D, Gulkesen H, Teber D, Rassweiler J (2005) Comparison of training modalities for performing laparoscopic radical prostatectomy: experience with 1000 patients. J Urol 174:673–678

Galli S, Simonato A, Bozzola A, Gregori A, Lissiani A, Scaburri A, Gaboardi F (2006) Oncologic outcome and continence recovery after laparoscopic radical prostatectomy: 3 years' follow-up in a "second generation center." Eur Urol 49(5):859–865

Geary ES, Dendinger TE, Freiha FS, Stamey TA (1995) Incontinence and vesical neck strictures following radical retropubic prostatectomy. Urology 45(6):1000–1006

Gettman M, Hoznek A, Salomon L, Katz R, Borkowski T, Antiphon P, Lobintiu A, Abbou C (2003) Laparoscopic radical prostatectomy: description of the extraperitoneal approach using the da Vinci robotic system. J Urol 170:416–419

Gill I, Zippe C (2001) Laparoscopic radical prostatectomies: technique. Urol Clin North Am 28:423–428

Goad JR, Scardino PT (1994) Modifications in the technique of radical retropubic prostatectomy to minimize blood loss. Urol Clin North Am 2:65–80

Goeman L, Salomon L, La De Taille A, Vordos D, Hoznek A, Yiou R, Abbou CC (2006) Long-term functional and oncological results after retroperitoneal laparoscopic prostatectomy according to a prospective evaluation of 550 patients. World J Urol 24:281–288

Gonzalgo ML, Pavlovich CP, Trock BJ, Link RE, Sullivan W, Su LM (2005). Classification and trends of perioperative morbidities following laparoscopic radical prostatectomy. J Urol. 174(1): 135–139

Graefen M (2006) The positive surgical margin after radical prostatectomy- Why do we still not really know what it means? Eur Urol 50:199–201

Graefen M, Walz J, Huland H (2006) Open retropubic nerve-sparing radical prostatectomy. Eur Urol 49:38–48

Guillonneau B, Cathelineau X, Barret E, Rozet F, Vallancien G (1999) Laparoscopic radical prostatectomy: technical and early oncological assessment of 40 operations. Eur Urol 36(1):14–20

Guillonneau B, Vallancien G (2000) Laparoscopic radical prostatectomy: the Montsouris technique. J Urol 63(6):1643–1649

Guillonneau B, Rozet F, Barret E, Cathelineau X, Vallancien G (2001) Laparoscopic radical prostatectomy: assessment after 240 procedures. Urol Clin North Am 28(1):189–202

Guillonneau B, Cathelineau X, Doublet JD et al. (2002a) Laparoscopic radical prostatectomy: assessment after 550 procedures. Crit Rev Oncol Hematol 43:123

Guillonneau B, Rozet F, Cathlineau X et al. (2002b) Perioperative complications of laparoscopic radical prostatectomy: the Montsouris 3-year experience. J Urol 167:51

Guillonneau B, el-Fettouh H, Baumert H, Cathelineau X, Doublet JD, Fromont G, Vallancien G (2003) Laparoscopic radical prostatectomy: oncological evaluation after 1,000 cases a Montsouris Institute. J Urol 169(4):1261–1266

Guilloneau B (2006) To demonstrate the benefits of laparoscopic radical prostatectomy? Eur Urol 50:1160–1162

Han M, Partin AW, Pound CR, Epstein JI, Walsh PC (2001) Long-term biochemical disease-free and cancer specific survival following anatomic radical retropubic prostatectomy. Urol Clin North Am 28:555–565

Hara I, Kawabata G, Miake H, Nakamura I, Hara S, Okada H, et al. (2003) Comparison of quality of life following laparoscopic and open prostatectomy for prostate cancer. J Urol 169:2045–2048

Harris MJ (2003) Radical perineal prostatectomy: cost efficient, outcome effective, minimally invasive prostate cancer management. Eur Urol 44:303–308

Hoznek A, Salomon L, Olsson LE, Antiphon P, Saint F, Cicco A, Chopin D, Abbou CC (2001) Laparoscopic radical prostatectomy. The Creteil experience. Eur Urol 40(1):38–45

Hoznek A, Antiphon P, Borkowski T, Gettman MT, Katz R, Salomon L, et al. (2003) Assessment of surgical technique and perioperative morbidity associated with extraperitoneal versus transperitoneal laparoscopic radical prostatectomy. Urology 61:617–622

Hull GW, Rabbani F, Abbas F, Wheeler TM, Kattan MW, Scardino PT (2002) Cancer control with radical prostatectomy alone in 1,000 consecutive patients. J Urol 167:528–534

Jacob F, Salomon L, Hoznek A, Bellot J, Antiphon P, Chopin DK, Abbou CC (2000) Laparoscopic radical prostatectomy: preliminary results. Eur Urol 37:615–620

Joseph J, Rosenbaum R, Madeb R et al. (2006) Robotic extraperitoneal radical prostatectomy: an alternative approach. J Urol 175:945–950

Kao TC, Cruess DF, Garner D, Foley J, Seay T, Friedrichs P, Thrasher JB, Mooneyhan RD, McLeod DG, Moul JW (2000) Multicenter patient self-reporting questionnaire on impotence, incontinence and stricture after radical prostatectomy. J Urol 163(3):870–871

Katz R, Borkowski T, Hoznek A, et al. (2003) Operative management of rectal injuries during laparoscopic radical prostatectomy. Urology 62:310

Kaul S, Bhandari A, Hemal A, Savera A, Shrivastava A, Menon M (2005) Robotic radical prostatectomy with preservation of the prostatic fascia: a feasibility study. Urology 66:1261–1265

Kirby R, Partin A, Feneley M, Parsons JK (2006) Prostate cancer: principles and practice. In: Robert PM and Arnauld V (eds) Chapter: anatomic considerations in radical prostatectomy. Informa Healthcare, Taylor & Francis, New York

Kleinhans B, Gerharz E, Melekos M, Weingartner K, Kalble T, Riedmiller H (1999) Changes of urodynamic findings after radical retropubic prostatectomy. Eur Urol 35(3):217–222

Leandri P, Rossignol G, Gautier JR, Ramon J (1992) Radical retropubic prostatectomy: morbidity and quality of life. Experience with 620 consecutive cases. J Urol 147(3 Pt 2):883–887

Lein M, Stibane I, Mansour R, Hege C, Roigas J, Wille A, Jung K, Kristiansen G, Schnorr D, Loening SA, Deger S (2006) Complications, urinary continence, and oncologic outcome of 1000 laparoscopic transperitoneal radical prostatectomies-experience at the Charite Hospital Berlin, Campus Mitte. Eur Urol 50(6):1278–82; discussion 1283–1284

Link RE, Su L-M, Sullivan W, Bhayani SB, Pavlovich CP (2005) Health related quality of life before and after laparoscopic radical prostatectomy. J Urol 173:175–179

Lotan Y, Cadeddu JA, Gettman MT (2004) The new economics of radical prostatectomy: cost comparison of open, laparoscopic and robot assisted techniques. J Urol 172(4 Pt 1):1431–1435

Matsunaga GS, Ahlering TE, Skarecky DW (2006) Update on Robotic Laparoscopic prostatectomy. TheScientificWorldJOURNAL 6:2542–2552

Menon M, Shrisvastava A, Tewari A, Sarle R, Hemal A, Peabody JO, Vallancien G (2002) Laparoscopic and robot assisted radical prostatectomy: establishment of a structured program and preliminary analysis of outcomes. J Urol 168: 945–949

Menon M, Tewari A, Peabody J (2003a) Vattikuti Institute prostatectomy: technique. J Urol 169(6):2289–2292

Menon M, Shrivastava A, Sarle R, Hemal A, Tewari A (2003b) Vattikuti Institute prostatectomy: a single team experience of 100 cases. J Endourol 17:785–790

Menon M, Tewari A, Peabody JO, Shrivastava A, Kaul S, Bhandari A, Hemal AK (2004) Vattikuti Institute prostatectomy, a technique of robotic radical prostatectomy for management of localized carcinoma of the prostate: experience of over 1100 cases. Urol Clin North Am 31(4):701–717

Menon M, Shrivastava A, Tewari A (2005) Laparoscopic radical prostatectomy: conventional and robotic. Urology 66 (5 Suppl):101–104

Menon M, Shrivastava A, Kaul S, Badani KK, Fumo M, Bhandari M, Peabody JO (2007) Vattikuti institute prostatectomy: contemporary technique and analysis of results. Eur Urol 51(3):648–658

Montorsi F, Salonia A, Suardi N, et al. (2005) Improving the preservation of the urethral sphincter and neurovascular bundles during open retropubic prostatectomy. Eur Urol 48:938–945

Omar AM, Townell N (2004) Laparoscopic radical prostatectomy a review of the literature and comparison with open techniques. Prostate Cancer Prostatic Dis 7:295–301

Ong AM, Su LM, Varkarakis I, Inagaki T, Link RE, Bhayani SB, Patriciu A, Crain B, Walsh PC (2004) Nerve sparing radical prostatectomy: Effects of hemostatic energy sources on the recovery of cavernous nerve function in a canine model. J Urol 172(4 pt 1):1318–1322

Palisaar RJ, Noldus J, Graefen M, Erbersdobler A, Haese A, Huland H (2005) Influence of nerve-sparing (NS) procedure during radical prostatectomy (RP) on margin status and biochemical failure. Eur Urol 47(2):176–184

Parker SL, Thong T, Bolden S, et al. (1996) Cancer statistics. CA Cancer J 46:5–67 2 t 1

Pasticier G, Rietbergen JB, Guillonneau B, Fromont G, Menon M, Vallancien G (2001) Robotically assisted laparoscopic radical prostatectomy: feasibility study in men. Eur Urol 40(1): 70–74

Patel VR, Tully AS, Holmes R, Lindsay J (2005) Robotic radical prostatectomy in the community setting: the learning curve and beyond: initial 200 cases. J Urol 174(1):269–272

Patel VR, Shah S, Arend D (2006) Histopathologic outcomes of Robotic Radical Prostatectomy. The Scientific World Journal 6:2566–2572

Perer E, Lee D, Ahlering T, Clayman R (2004) Robotic revelation: laparoscopic radical prostatectomy by non-laparoscopic surgeon. J Am Coll Surg 197:693–696

Poulakis V, Dillenburg W, Moeckel M, de Vries R, Witzsch U, Zumbe ´J, Rassweiler J, Becht E (2005) Laparoscopic radical prostatectomy: prospective evaluation of the learning curve. Eur Urol 47:167–175

Rabbani F, Patel MI, Scardino PT (2004) Time course of recovery of potency after bilateral nerve sparing radical prostatectomy. J Urol (suppl 171):310, Abstract [1178]

Raboy A, Ferzli G, Albert P (1997) Initial experience with extraperitoneal endoscopic radical retropubic prostatectomy. Urology 50(6):849–853

Rassweiler J, Binder J, Frede T (2001a) Robotic and telesurgery: will they change the future. Curr Opinion in Urology 11:309–320

Rassweiler J, Sentker L, Seemann O, Hatziger M, Stock C, Frede T (2001b) Heilbronn laparoscopic radical prostatectomy: technique and results after 100 cases. Eur Urol 40:54–64

Rassweiler J, Senkter L, Seeman O, et al. (2001c) Laparoscopic radical prostatectomy with the Heilbronn technique: an analysis of the first 180 cases. Eur Urol 166:2101

Rassweiler J, Seemann O, Schulze M, Teber D, Hatzinger M, Frede T (2003) Laparoscopic versus open radical prostatectomy: a comparative study at a single institution. J Urol 169(5): 1689–1693

Rassweiler J, Schulze M, Teber D, Seemann O, Frede T (2004) Laparoscopic radical prostatectomy: functional and oncological outcomes. Curr Opin Urol 14:75–82

Rassweiler J, Hruza M, Teber D, Schulze M, Stock C, Frede T (2005a) Quality of life following laparoscopic radical prostatectomy: the Heilbronn experience. Eur Urol 4(3) Suppl: 246 [Abstract 973]

Rassweiler J, Schulze M, Teber D, Marrero R, Seemann O, Rumpelt J, Frede T (2005b) Laparoscopic radical prostatectomy with the Heilbronn technique: oncological results in the first 500 patients. J Urol 173(3):761–764

Rassweiler J (2006) Intrafascial nerve-sparing laparoscopic radical prostatectomy: Do we really preserve relevant fibers? Eur Urol 49:955–957

Rassweiler J, Hruza M, Teber D, Su LM (2006a) Laparoscopic and robotic assisted radical prostatectomy- Critical analysis of the results. Eur Urol 49:612–624

Rassweiler J, Stolzenburg J, Sulser T, Deger S, Zumbe J, Hofmockel G, John H, Janetschek G, Fehr JL, Hatzinger M, Probst M, Rothenberger KH, Poulakis V, Truss M, Popken G, Westphal J, Alles U, Fornara P (2006b) Laparoscopic radical prostatectomy–the experience of the German Laparoscopic Working Group. Eur Urol 49(1):113–119

Remzi M, Klingler HC, Tinzl MV, Fong YK, Lobe M, Kiss B, et al. (2005) Morbidity of laparoscopic extraperitoneal versus transperitoneal radical prostatectomy versus open retropubic radical radical prostatectomy. Eur Urol 48:83–89

Roumeguere T, Bollens R, Vanden Bossche M, Rochet D, Bialek D, Hoffman P, Quackels T, Damoun A, Wespes E, Schulman CC, Zlotta AR (2003) Radical prostatectomy: a prospective comparison of oncological and functional results between open and laparoscopic approaches. World J Urol 20(6):360–652

Rozet F, Harmon J, Cathelineau X, Barret E, Vallancien G (2006) Robot-assisted versus pure laparoscopic radical prostatectomy. World J Urol 24(2):171–179

Ruiz L, Salomon L, Hoznek A, Vordos D, Yiou R, de la Taille A, et al. (2004) Comparison of early oncologic results of laparoscopic radical prostatectomy by extraperitoneal versus transperitoneal approach. Eur Urol 46:50–56

Salomon L, Levrel O, de la Taille A, Anastasiadis AG, Saint F, Zaki S, Vordos D, Cicco A, Olsson LE, Hoznek A, Chopin D, Abbou CC (2002) Radical prostatectomy by the retropubic, perineal and laparoscopic approach: 12 years of experience in one center. Eur Urol 42(2):104–111

Salomon L, Saint F, Anastasiadis G, Sebe P, Chopin D, Abbou CC (2003) Combined reporting of cancer control and functional results of radical prostatectomy. Eur Urol 44:656–660

Salomon L, Sebe P, De la Taille A, Vordos D, Hoznek A, Yiou R, Chopin D, Abbou CC (2004) Open versus laparoscopic radical prostatectomy: part I. BJU Int 94(2):238–243

Samadi D, Levinson A, Hakimi A, Shabsigh R, Benson MC (2007) From proficiency to expert, when does the learning curve for robotic-assisted prostatectomies plateau? The Columbia University experience. World J Urol

Scardino PT (2005) Continuing refinements in radical prostatectomy: more evidence that technique matters. J Urol 173(2):338–339

Schuessler WW, Kavoussi LR, Clayman RV, Vancaille TH (1992) Laparoscopic radical prostatectomy: initial case report [abstract 130]. J Urol 147:246A

Schuessler W, Schulman P, Clayman R, Kavoussi L (1997) Laparoscopic radical prostatectomy: initial short-term experience. Urology 50:854–857

Slawin KM, Guariguata L (2006) The influence of increasing experience and surgical technique on surgical margin status in patients undergoing open and robotic prostatectomy by a single surgeon. AUA abstract [1164]

Smith Jr JA (2004) Robotically assisted laparoscopic prostatectomy: an assessment of its contemporary role in the surgical management of localized cancer. Am J Surg 188(Suppl):635–675

Söderdahl DW, Davis JW, Schellhammer PF, Given RW, Lynch DF, Shaves M, et al. (2005) Prospective longitudinal comparative study of health related quality of life in patients undergoing invasive treatments for localized prostate cancer. J Endourol 19:318–326

Stanford JL, Feng Z, Hamilton AS, Gilliland FD, Stephenson RA, Eley JW, Albertsen PC, Harlan LC, Potosky AL (2000) Urinary and sexual function after radical prostatectomy for clinically localized prostate cancer: the Prostate Cancer Outcomes Study. JAMA 283:354

Steiner MS (2000) Continence-preserving anatomical radical retropubic prostatectomy. Urology 55:427–435

Stolzenburg JU, Do M, Pfeiffer H, Konig F, Aedtner B, Dorschner W (2002) The endoscopic extraperitoneal radical prostatectomy (EERPE): technique and initial experience. World J Urol 20(1):48–55

Stolzenburg JU, Truss MC, Do M, Rabenalt R, Pfeiffer H, Dunzinger M, Aedtner B, Stief CG, Jonas U, Dorschner W (2003) Evolution of endoscopic extraperitoneal radical prostatectomy (EERPE)-technical improvements and development of a nerve-sparing, potency-preserving approach. World J Urol 21(3):147–152

Stolzenburg JU, Rabenalt R, Do M, Ho K, Dorschner W, Waldkirch E, Jonas U, Schutz A, Horn L, Truss MC (2005) Endoscopic extraperitoneal radical prostatectomy: oncological and functional results after 700 procedures. J Urol 174(4 Pt 1): 1271–1275

Stolzenburg JU, Rabenalt R, Do M, Horn LC, Liatsikos EN (2006a) Modular training for residents with no prior experience with open pelvic surgery in endoscopic extraperitoneal radical prostatectomy. Eur Urol 49:491–500

Stolzenburg JU, Rabenalt R, Do M, Tannapfel A, Truss MC, Liatsikos EN (2006b) Nerve-sparing endoscopic extraperitoneal radical prostatectomy: University of Leipzig technique. J Endourol 20(11):925–929

Stolzenburg JU, Rabenalt R, Do M, Truss MC, Burchardt M, Herrmann TR, Schwalenberg T, Kallidonis P, Liatsikos EN (2007) Endoscopic extraperitoneal radical prostatectomy. The University of Leipzig experience of 1,300 cases. World J Urol 25(1):45–51

Su LM, Link RE, Bhayani SB, Sullivan W, Pavlovich CP (2004) Nerve-sparing laparoscopic radical prostatectomy: Replicating the open surgical technique. Urology 64:123–127

Sullivan LD, Weir MJ, Kinahan JF, Taylor DL (2000) A comparison of the relative merits of radical perineal and radical retropubic prostatectomy. BJU Int 85(1):95–100

Sulser T, Guilloneau B, Vallancien G, Gastion R, Piechaud T, Türk I (2001) Complications and initial experience with 1228 laparoscopic radical prostatectomies at 6 European centers. J Urol 165(Suppl):150

Takenaka A, Leung RA, Fujisawa M, Tewari AK (2006) Anatomy of autonomic nerve component in the male pelvis: the new concept from a perspective for robotic nerve sparing radical prostatectomy. World J Urol 24(2):136–143

Takenaka A, Tewari AK, Leung RA, Bigelow K, El-Tabey N, Murakami G, Fujisawa M (2007) Preservation of the puboprostatic collar and puboperineoplasty for early recovery of urinary continence after robotic prostatectomy: anatomic basis and preliminary outcomes. Eur Urol 51(2):433–440

Talcott JA, Rieker P, Propert KJ, Clark JA, Wishnow KI, Loughlin KR, Richie JP, Kantoff PW (1997) Patient-reported impotence and incontinence after nerve-sparing radical prostatectomy. J Natl Cancer Inst 89:1117–1123

Tewari A, Paebody J, Sarle R, Balakrishnan G, Hemal A, Shrivastava A, Menon M (2002) Technique of da Vinci robot-assisted anatomic radical prostatectomy. Urology 60:569–572

Tewari A, Srivasatava A, Menon M (2003) Members of the VIP Team. prospective comparison of radical retropubic and robot-assisted prostatectomy: experience in one institution. BJU Int 92(3):205–210

Tewari A, Takenaka A, Mtui E, Horninger W, Peschel R, Bartsch G, Vaughan ED (2006) The proximal neurovascular plate and the tri-zonal neural architecture around the prostate gland: importance in the athermal robotic technique of nerve-sparing prostatectomy. BJU Int 98(2):314–323

Tsuboi T, Ohori M, Kuroiwa K, Reuter VE, Kattan MW, Eastham JA, Scardino PT (2005) Is intraoperative frozen section analysis an efficient way to reduce positive surgical margins? Urology 66(6):1287–1291

Touijer K, Kuroiwa K, Vickers A, Reuter VE, Hricak H, Scardino PT, Guillonneau B (2006) Impact of a multidisciplinary continuous quality improvement program on the positive surgical margin rate after laparoscopic radical prostatectomy. Eur Urol 49(5):853–858

Türk I, Deger S, Winkelmann B, Schonberger B, Loening SA (2001) Laparoscopic radical prostatectomy. Technical aspects and experience with 125 cases. Eur Urol 40(1):46–53

Wagner A, Link R, Pavlovich C, Sullivan W, Su L (2006) Use of a validated quality of life questionnaire to assess sexual function following laparoscopic radical prostatectomy. Int J Impot Res 18(1):69–76

Walsh PC, Donker PJ (1982) Impotence following radical prostatectomy: insight into etiology and prevention. J Urol 128(3): 492–497

Walsh PC, Lepor H, Eggleston JD (1983) Radical prostatectomy with preservation of sexual function: anatomical and pathological considerations. Prostate 157(5):1760–1767

Walsh PC (1998) Anatomic radical prostatectomy: evolution of the surgical technique. J Urol 160(6 Pt 2):2418–2424

Walsh PC, Marschke P, Ricker D, Burnett AL (2000) Patient reported urinary continence and sexual function after anatomic radical prostatectomy. Urology 55:58–61

Wieder JA, Soloway MS (1998) Incidence, etiology, location, prevention and treatment of positive surgical margins after radical prostatectomy for prostate cancer. J Urol 160(2):299–315

Wolfram M, Brautigam R, Engl T, Bentas W, Heitkamp S, Ostwald M, Kramer W, Binder J, Blaheta R, Jonas D, Beecken WD (2003) Robotic-assisted laparoscopic radical prostatectomy: the Frankfurt technique. World J Urol 21(3):128–132

Zorn KC, Gofrit ON, Orvieto MA, Mikhail AA, Zagaja GP, Shalhav AL (2007) Robotic-assisted laparoscopic prostatectomy: functional and pathologic outcomes with interfascial nerve preservation. Eur Urol 51:755–763

Chapter 5
Robotic-Assisted Radical Cystectomy

P. Dasgupta, P. Rimington, A.K. Hemal, and M.S. Khan

Abstract: Robotic-assisted radical cystectomy (RARC) is an evolving procedure which combines the minimally invasive benefits of laparoscopy and the enhanced dexterity and vision of robotics. Over 150 of these have been performed worldwide in selected centers. Although the blood loss, hospital stay, and recovery are shorter than open surgery, operative times are longer. In nonrandomized comparisons, the complications appear to be lower than open and laparoscopic radical cystectomy. Actuarial and recurrence-free survivals at 3.5 years are 95 and 90%, respectively. A single port site recurrence has been reported.

Keywords: Robotics, Cystectomy, Urinary diversion, Oncologic outcome

5.1. Introduction

Although randomized controlled trials are lacking, radical cystectomy/anterior exenteration is currently regarded as the gold standard for managing invasive bladder cancer,extensive uncontrollable superficial cancer and refractory carcinoma in situ (CIS). At specialized centers the 5-year recurrence free survival for muscle invasive disease is 56–73% (Madersbacher et al. 2003). Herr et al. have proposed optimum standards for

P. Dasgupta (ed.), *Robotic Urological Surgery in Clinical Practice*,   113
DOI: 10.1007/978-1-84800-243-2_5,
© Springer-Verlag London Limited 2008

this procedure. These include 10% positive surgical margins overall and 15% in patients with T3 & T4 tumors. The median number of lymph nodes retrieved should be 10–14 (Herr et al. 2004). Although open radical cystectomy (ORC) has become safer in expert hands, it remains a formidable procedure with a complication rate of around 30–50%. Excessive bowel handling, fluid loss, and opiates can lead to prolonged ileus. In spite of improvements in surgical techniques blood loss during ORC is often significant. The hospital stay is consequently quite prolonged with 18–21 days quoted as the UK average (Nuttall et al. 2005).

Urologists experienced in advanced laparoscopy have reported promising results of laparoscopic radical cystectomy (LRC) in the hope of reducing patient morbidity. Within our own group LRC is performed by a team consisting of two experienced urologists to reduce surgical fatigue (Rimington and Dasgupta 2004). The procedure is sometimes difficult due to reduced maneuverability of laparoscopic instruments in the pelvis. The complication rate of LRC can be high even in expert hands. The overall complications during hospital stay and after discharge have been up to 46 and 19%, respectively (Haber and Gill 2007). Another large LRC series of 84 patients showed that the complication rate can be reduced to 18% which is better than reported in most series of ORC (Cathelineau et al. 2005). The da Vinci™ system (Intuitive Surgical, California) has the potential to overcome some of the technical difficulties of LRC. We published the first UK experience with this system (Dasgupta et al. 2005) and now review the oncologic and functional outcomes of robotic-assisted radical cystectomy (RARC). At the time of writing >150 procedures have been performed worldwide.

5.2. Surgical Technique

The Guy's technique is derived from ORC and LRC and has evolved over 4 years (Raychaudhuri et al. 2006). Patients

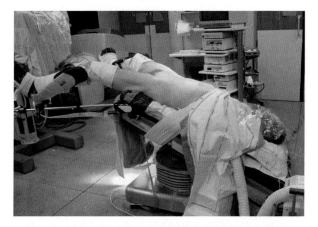

FIGURE 5.1 Position of patient during robotic cystectomy.

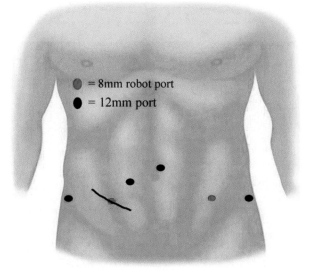

FIGURE 5.2 Schematic diagram of port positioning.

are given clear fluids orally, an enema the day before their operation and overnight intravenous normal saline to prevent dehydration. This is part of an enhanced recovery program derived from colorectal surgery where formal bowel preparation is deliberately avoided. Intravenous cefuroxime and metronidazole and subcutaneous low molecular weight heparin are administered perioperatively. Patients above 60 are digitalized as recommended by urologists experienced in open cystectomy, to prevent atrial fibrillation (Stein and Skinner 2004). They are placed in the extended lithotomy position with a 45° Trendelenburg tilt (Fig. 5.1). A disposable sigmoidoscope is introduced per rectum in male and a methylene blue-soaked swab per vaginam in female patients. After sterile catheterization, a six-port transperitoneal approach is used as previously described (Hemal et al. 2004) (Fig. 5.2). The ports are usually placed in a fan-shaped configuration (Fig. 5.3). The procedure involves three surgeons—one at the console and one on each side of the patient. A fourth robotic arm can be used in place of the left side assistant.

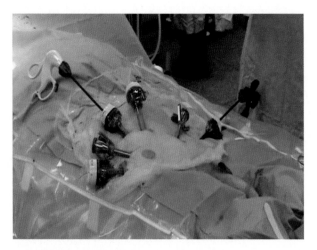

FIGURE 5.3 Port positioning.

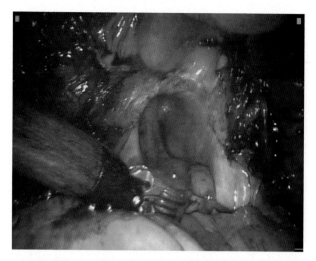

FIGURE 5.4 Posterior dissection.

5.2.1. Posterior Dissection

The ureters are mobilized in the pelvis while keeping adequate tissue around them so as not to compromise their vascularity. The distal ends are clipped and cut and sent for frozen section analysis. An inverted U-shaped incision is made in the peritoneum of the cul-de-sac (Pouch of Douglas) (Fig. 5.4). The posterior layer of Denonvillier's fascia is then incised in the midline and the plane between the rectum and the prostate developed. In patients wishing to preserve potency, diathermy is avoided at the tips of the seminal vesicles to avoid injury to the pelvic plexus. In females, the ovarian vessels are controlled with Hem-o-lok clips (Weck Closure Systems, NC, USA) and divided. The plane between the rectum and uterus is developed and the uterine arteries controlled with Hem-o-loks.

5.2.2. Lateral Dissection

Dissection is continued medial to the external iliac veins to carefully preserve the obturator nerves and expose the lateral

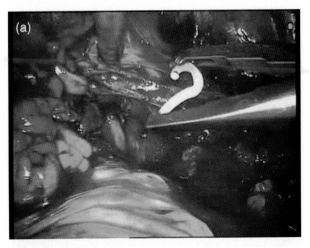

FIGURE 5.5A Control of lateral pedicles of the bladder with clips.

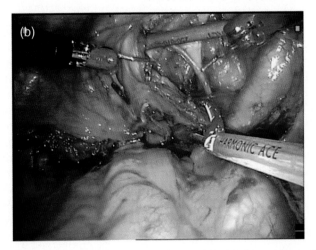

FIGURE 5.5B Control of lateral pedicles of the bladder with staples.

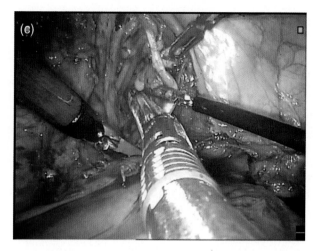

FIGURE 5.5C Control of lateral pedicles of the bladder with harmonic scalpel.

pelvic wall. This delineates the lateral pedicles to the bladder (and uterus in females). We initially used Hem-o-lok clips for control of the lateral pedicles but subsequently switched to an Endopath™ ATW45 linear stapler (Ethicon Endosurgery, Livingston, UK). This was prompted by our perception that blood loss was somewhat higher with clips. Currently, an ACE Harmonic™ scalpel (Ethicon Endosurgery, Livingston, UK) seems to be the most efficient (Fig. 5.5a–c) for this purpose. It is also more cost-effective ~£300 for harmonic as opposed to £1200 for staplers since multiple firings of cartridges are required.

5.2.3. Anterior Dissection

The bladder is filled with 200 ml of formol-saline for easy identification and dropped by an inverted U incision to include the urachus. The endopelvic fascia is opened and the dorsal vein controlled by a stitch. Nerve sparing is performed in potent patients. The dorsal vein complex and urethra are cut and a clip placed on the specimen side of the urethra to prevent any spillage. The distal urethral margin is sent for frozen section. In females the urethra is dissected fully to the external meatus. The posterior vaginal fornix is opened. The previously placed methylene blue swab becomes visible indicating that the correct plane had been entered. The lateral vaginal walls are transected. The cystectomy specimens are placed in a 15-mm EndoCatch II^{TM} bag (Tyco Healthcare, Hampshire, UK) for later retrieval. Leakage of carbon dioxide from the vagina is reduced by a water-proof dressing applied externally. The vagina is then closed longitudinally by continuous intracorporeal suturing.

5.2.4. Lymphadenectomy, Transposition of Left Ureter

Using robotic bipolar forceps and scissors, careful bilateral lymphadenectomy is performed. The limits of the dissection are the genitofemoral nerve laterally, the bifurcation of the common iliac artery proximally and the node of Cloquet distally. Care is taken to preserve the obturator nerve. The da Vinci^{TM} S-HD gives better quadrantic access and it is possible to extend the lymph node dissection to the aortic bifurcation with this new system. The lymph nodal packs are placed in separately marked laparoscopic sacks. An Endoloop^{TM} (Ethicon Endo-surgery, Livingston, UK) is applied on the distal end of the left ureter which is then transposed under the sigmoid mesocolon to the left by pulling the Endoloop through. The distal ends of the ureters are held together with a laparoscopic grasper introduced through the left-sided 5-mm assistant port.

5.2.5. Urinary Diversion

It is easier and quicker to perform urinary diversions extracorporeally although complete robotic-assisted intracorporeal diversion has been reported. For ileal conduits a 15-cm segment of ileum about 15-cm proximal to the ileo-cecal junction is held in laparoscopic graspers introduced through the most lateral right-sided 10-mm port. The robot is undocked. The previously bagged bladder and lymph nodal specimens are extracted through a 5–7-cm incision (Fig. 5.6). In thin patients this is an appendix muscle-splitting incision made by extending a lateral port while in overweight patients (BMI >30 kg/m^2) a subumbilical midline incision is preferred for easier left ureteric access. The graspers holding the ureters and ileal segment are brought to the surface through this incision. The ileal loop is isolated on its mesentery, bowel continuity restored with staplers and the mesenteric window closed. Ureteroileal anastomosis is performed over 8F feeding tubes by a Wallace I technique. The distal end of the conduit is fashioned as a stoma at a previously marked site on the abdominal wall. A sump drain is introduced into the conduit to prevent any anastomotic pressure and leak from subsequent stomal edema. Studer

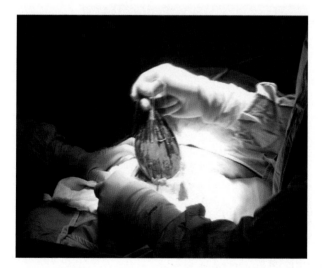

FIGURE 5.6 Specimen extraction in laparoscopic sack.

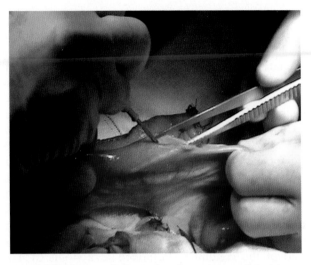

FIGURE 5.7 Studer pouch formation through a small incision.

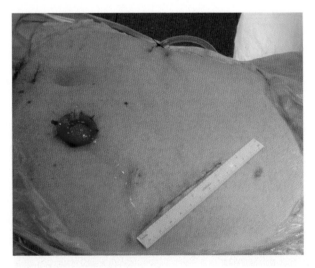

FIGURE 5.8 Postoperative wounds.

pouches are created through lower midline incisions and anastomosed to the urethral stump by six robotically placed 3–0 Monocryl sutures (Fig. 5.7). Alternatively, a continuous 3–0 Monocryl anastomosis can be performed as in radical prostatectomy, after redocking the robot. A 20 F drain is placed in the pelvis. The port sites and wounds are closed with absorbable sutures (Fig. 5.8). A liter of icodextrin (Adept, ML Pharmaceuticals,Warrington, UK) is instilled into the abdomen and drained after an hour to reduce the risk of bowel adhesions.

5.3. Postoperative Care

All patients are electively managed in an overnight recovery or high dependency unit immediately after the operation. The naso-gastric tube is removed and oral liquids started as tolerated. Early mobilization and chest physiotherapy are encouraged. Most patients are discharged with their pelvic drains and ureteric catheters in situ which are removed at 3 weeks. Patients are seen again at 6 weeks, have an abdominal ultrasound at 3 months, CT scans at 6 months and then at 6-monthly intervals. At these visits they also undergo clinical examination and assessment of serum hemoglobin, electrolytes, creatinine, chloride, and bicarbonate.

5.4. Outcomes of RARC

RARC and urinary diversion was initially reported in 2003 (Menon et al. 2003). Similar to LRC, it involved a six-port transperitoneal approach. The procedure was performed in three stages: initially pelvic lymphadenectomy and cystoprostatectomy, secondly extracorporeal formation of a neobladder, and thirdly intracorporeal urethroneovesical anastomosis following redocking of the robot. The operative times ranged from 260–308 min depending on whether an ileal conduit or orthotopic neobladder was formed. Blood loss was <150 mls and surgical margins were clear in all cases. One patient had N1 disease. Long-term oncologic or functional results were not reported although a port-site metastasis was subsequently mentioned (El-Tabey and Shoma 2005). Around the same time Beeken et al. described robotic cystectomy and intracorporeal Hautmann orthotopic neobladder with an operating time of 8.5 hours and a blood loss of 200 ml (Beecken et al. 2003), whilst Balaji et al. successfully performed robotic-assisted totally intracorporeal laparoscopic ileal conduit urinary diversion in three patients (Balaji et al. 2004) with operative time of 630–830 min and a hospital stay of 5–10 days. The longest operative time was in one patient who underwent concomitant RARC. Menon's group subsequently refined the robotic technique for women with preservation of the uterus and vagina (Menon et al. 2004). Other authors have excluded patients with prior extensive abdominal surgery, pelvic irradiation, neoadjuvant chemotherapy, and extravesical mass on CT from RARC (Miller and Theodorescu 2005), making a selection bias quite likely. Guru et al. reported their early results on 20 RARC with average age of 70 and BMI of 26 kg/m^2. The mean operative duration was 442 min, blood loss 555 ml, and hospital stay of 10 days. The procedure was unsuccessful in a patient with fixed pelvic mass and another needed conversion to open surgery as the patient could not tolerate the Trendelenburg position. There were three bowel obstructions, one of whom died of sepsis and one readmission with pyelonephritis. Thus, the overall complication rate was 20%. One patient had positive vaginal margins and 9 of 26 lymph nodes were positive (Guru et al. 2007). In 30 patients at Guy's the operative time was between 5.5–8 hours depending on whether an ileal conduit or Studer pouch was created, estimated blood loss 200 ml, and hospital stay either 1 week for the conduits or 2 weeks for the pouches. One patient needed blood transfusion due to bleeding from an inferior epigastric artery and one patient with a large urethral adenocarcinoma needed a colostomy for rectal injury. Delayed functional complications occurred in three patients. One patient with a Studer pouch developed a neovesico-urethral stricture which needed urethral dilatation. Another developed a left upper ureteric stricture at 6 months. This was assumed to be malignant and hence treated with nephroureterectomy. The final pathology was that of a benign inflammatory stricture. A third patient needed repair of an incisional hernia at 12 months. Serum creatinine levels were maintained in all patients. Three of four previously potent male patients who underwent nerve sparing were potent with Tadalafil.

The operation has also been performed in patients without cancer. Two men, 41 and 38 years old, with complete post-traumatic C7–C8 quadriplegia underwent total intracorporeal cystoprostatectomy and ileal conduit urinary diversion with robotic assistance. The procedures were completed without open conversion. The total surgical time was 9.25 and 6.75 hours, respectively. There were no intraoperative complications. In the postoperative period, both patients had complications (pulmonary and urinary infections) that were treated medically. The postoperative hospital stay was 13 days (Hubert et al. 2006).

5.5. Comparison of ORC and RARC

Rhee et al. compared 23 ORC to seven RARC and found that although blood loss was lower for RARC, four of seven patients (57%) needed transfusion. The operative duration was 638 min for RARC vs. 507 min for ORC and hospital stay 11 and 13 days, respectively (Rhee et al. 2006). In another study of 37 patients, 24 (64.9%) had ORC and 13 (29.7%) were treated with RARC. RARC resulted in significantly lower blood loss, hospital stay, and longer operating time compared with ORC. Four (16.7%) perioperative complications occurred in the open group compared with two (15.4%) in the robotic group (Galich et al. 2006). Pruthi and Wallen compared 20 men undergoing RARC and extracorporeal urinary diversion to 24 matched men who underwent ORC. Mean operative time for RARC was 6.1 hours as opposed to

3.8 hours for ORC. Mean blood loss was significantly less for RARC. On surgical pathology 14 RARC cases were pT2 or less, four were pT3, and two were N+. There were no positive surgical margins. A mean of 19 lymph nodes was removed. Mean time to flatus and bowel movement was significantly shorter than in men undergoing ORC. There were six postoperative complications (30%) in five patients (Pruthi and Wallen 2007). Likewise, Wang et al. compared 20 ORC and 33 RARC patients and found similar complication rates (24% open, 21% robotic). The open cohort had more patients with extravesical disease (57 vs. 28%) and nodal metastasis (34 vs. 19%), although this may be a reflection of small sample size. There were three patients in the open group and two in the robotic with positive margins. The median number of lymph nodes removed was similar between groups (Wang et al. 2008).

5.6. Comparison of ORC, LRC, and RARC

Thirty age-matched patients (ten in each group) had ORC, LRC, or RARC and ileal conduit diversion by three surgeons (Table 5.1). RARC and LRC took longer than ORC but were associated with less blood loss and quicker recovery. Hospital stay was shortest for RARC, which also had the lowest complication rate (Elhage et al. 2007a).

5.7. Oncologic Outcomes

For RARC to stand the test of time, the oncologic outcomes have to be equivalent to ORC and LRC. In their series of 1054 patients undergoing ORC, Stein et al. reported recurrence-free survival at 5 and 10 years of 68 and 66%, respectively (Stein et al. 2001). The recurrence-free survival appears to be worse for patients with stage >pT2N0 (Madersbacher et al. 2003). On the basis of their results in ten LRC patients, five of whom died, Simonato et al. reported poorer

TABLE 5.1 Comparison of ORC, LRC, RARC

Op	Op time (mins)	Blood loss (mls)	Complication (%)	Hosp stay (days)	Recovery (weeks)	Oncologic follow-up
ORC	325	1300	60	16	8	60% RFS@5 yr
LRC	345	350	50	16	3	60% RFS@4 yr
RARC	365	150	20	10.5	4	90% RFS@3 yr

Note: RFS = Recurrence-free survival

oncologic outcomes with LRC compared to ORC (Simonato et al. 2005). In a recent study of 37 patients undergoing LRC, followed-up for up to 5 years, Haber and Gill reported actuarial overall and recurrence-free survival of 63 and 92%, respectively. However, only eight patients had completed 5 years of follow-up and oncologic data was not available in seven patients. Assuming that all these seven patients had died from metastatic disease, the recalculated 5-year overall and cancer-specific survival were 58 and 68%, respectively. The outcomes were poorer in those with concomitant CIS, extraorgan disease, and nodal metastasis. Patients having extended laparoscopic lymph node dissection had slightly better cancer specific survival compared to those having a limited template lymphadenectomy, although not reaching statistical significance (Haber and Gill 2007). With strict adherence to oncologic principles during RARC to prevent spillage of cancer cells, we reported 100% overall and recurrence-free survival at 2 years (Dasgupta et al. 2007). At a maximum follow-up of 3.5 years, the actuarial overall and recurrence-free survival, were 95 and 90%, respectively. A median of 16 (6–28) lymph nodes were removed. In our patient group, 10% had lymph nodal disease, 10% incidental prostate cancer, and 10% prostatic urethral CIS. There were no positive margins, no local pelvic recurrences, and no port-site metastasis. Lymph node metastasis, higher grade and concomitant CIS were predictors of poor medium-term outcome.

5.8. Quality of Life and Patient Satisfaction

Using quality of life questionnaires Guru et al. found time to normal activity to be 4 weeks, time to driving 6 weeks, and time to strenuous activity 10 weeks (Guru et al. 2007). Using the SF-8 validated questionnaire we found no change in physical quality of life scores at 6 weeks after RARC but significantly better mental scores (Fig. 5.9). Patient satisfaction was high (median 30 out of a maximum of 32 on a validated client satisfaction-8 survey; range 27–32). We found that 93% of

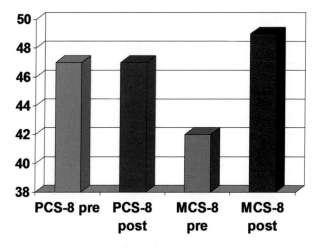

FIGURE 5.9 Assessment of physical and mental quality of life after robotic cystectomy.

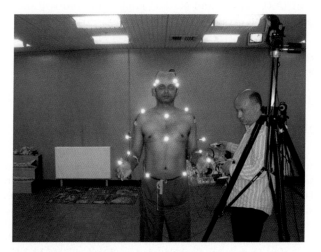

FIGURE 5.10 Assessment of surgical fatigue by motion analysis in a gait laboratory (Courtesy of: Adam Shortland).

patients read and understood the patient information leaflet provided and 60% elected to watch a robotic patient information video. This had been screened by the British Broadcasting Corporation (BBC) after appropriate patient consent.

5.9. Ergonomics

One of the advantages of RARC over ORC and LRC may be reduced surgical fatigue during a long procedure (Elhage et al. 2007b). This has been studied using motion analysis and EMG recordings in a gait lab (Fig. 5.10).

5.10. Conclusions

The medium-term surgical, oncologic, and functional outcomes of RARC are encouraging. A randomized controlled trial of ORC, LRC, and RARC is planned and will include detailed health economic modeling.

Acknowledgments Guy's and St. Thomas' Charity, British Urological Foundation

References

Balaji KC, Yohannes P, McBride CL, Oleynikov D, Hemstreet GP 3rd (2004) Feasibility of robot-assisted totally intracorporeal laparoscopic ileal conduit urinary diversion: Initial results of a single institutional pilot study. Urology 63:51–55

Beecken WD, Wolfram M, Engl T et al. (2003) Robotic-assisted Laparoscopic Radical Cystectomy and Intra-abdominal Formation of an Orthotopic Ileal Neobladder. Eur Urol 44:337–339

Cathelineau X, Arroyo C, Rozet F, Barret E, Vallancien G (2005) Laparoscopic assisted radical cystectomy: the Montsouris experience after 84 cases. Eur Urol 47:780–784

Dasgupta P, Hemal A, Rose K, Guy's and St. Thomas' Robotics Group (2005) Robotic urology in the UK: establishing a programme and emerging role. BJU Int 95:723–724

Dasgupta P, Rimington P, Murphy D et al. (2007) Robot-assisted radical cystectomy for bladder cancer and 2 year follow-up. BJU Int 99S1:P62

Elhage O, Keegan J, Varma P et al. (2007a) A comparative analysis of open, laparoscopic and robotic radical cystectomy for bladder cancer. J Endourol 21(S1):142A

Elhage O, Murphy D, Challacombe B, Shortland A, Dasgupta P (2007b) Ergonomics in minimally invasive surgery. Int J Clin Pract 61:186–188

El-Tabey NA, Shoma AM (2005) Port site metastases after robot-assisted laparoscopic radical cystectomy. Urology 66:1110

Galich A, Sterrett S, Nazemi T et al. (2006) Comparative analysis of early perioperative outcomes following radical cystectomy by either the robotic or open method. JSLS 10:145–150

Guru KA, Kim HL, Piacente PM, Mohler JL (2007) Robot-assisted radical cystectomy and pelvic lymph node dissection: initial experience at Roswell Park Cancer Institute. Urology 69:469–74

Haber G-P, Gill IS (2007) Laparoscopic radical cystectomy for cancer: oncological outcomes at up to 5 years. BJU Int 100:137–142

Hemal AK, Eun D, Tewari A, Menon M (2004) Nuances in the optimum placement of ports in pelvic and upper urinary tract surgery using the da Vinci robot. Urol Clin North Am 31:683–92, viii

Herr H, Lee C, Chang S, Lerner S for the bladder cancer collaborative group (2004) Standardization of radical cystectomy and pelvic lymph node dissection for bladder cancer. A collaborative group report. J Urol 171:1823–1828

Hubert J, Chammas M, Larre S et al. (2006) Initial experience with successful totally robotic laparoscopic cystoprostatectomy and ileal conduit construction in tetraplegic patients: report of two cases. J Endourol 20:139–143

Madersbacher S, Hochreiter W, Burkhard F et al. (2003) Radical cystectomy for bladder cancer today—a homogeneous series without neoadjuvant therapy. J Clin Oncol 21:690–696

Menon M, Hemal A, Tewari A et al. (2003) Nerve-sparing robot-assisted radical cystoprostatectomy and urinary diversion. BJU Int 92:232–236

Menon M, Hemal AK, Tewari A et al. (2004) Robot-assisted Radical Cystectomy and Urinary Diversion in Female Patients: Technique with Preservation of the Uterus and Vagina. J Am Coll Surg 198:386–393

Miller NL, Theodorescu D (2006) Status of robotic cystectomy in 2005. World J Urol 24:180–187

Nuttall MC, van der Meulen J, McIntosh G, Gillatt D, Emberton M (2005) Changes in patient characteristics and outcomes for radical cystectomy in England. BJU Int 95:513–516

Pruthi RS, Wallen EM (2007) Robotic assisted laparoscopic radical cystoprostatectomy: operative and pathological outcomes. J Urol 178(3 Pt 1):814–818

Raychaudhuri B, Khan MS, Challacombe B, Rimington P, Dasgupta P (2006) Minimally invasive radical cystectomy. BJU Int 98: 1064–1067

Rhee JJ, Lebeau S, Smolkin M, Theodorescu D (2006) Radical cystectomy with ileal conduit diversion: early prospective evaluation of the impact of robotic assistance. BJU Int 96:1059–1063

Rimington P, Dasgupta P (2004) Laparoscopic and robotic radical cystectomy. BJU Int 93:460–461

Simonato A, Gregori A, Lissiani A et al. (2005) Laparoscopic radical cystoprostatectomy: our experience in a consecutive series of 10 patients with a 3 years follow-up. Eur Urol 47:785–790

Stein JP, Lieskovsky G, Cote R et al. (2001) Radical cystectomy in the treatment of invasive bladder cancer: long-term results in 1054 patients. J Clin Oncol 19:666–675

Stein JP, Skinner DG (2004) Surgical atlas radical cystectomy. BJU Int 94:197–221

Wang GJ, Barocas DA, Raman JD et al. (2008) Robotic vs open radical cystectomy: prospective comparison of perioperative outcomes and pathological measures of early oncological efficacy. BJU Int 101:89–93

Chapter 6
Robotic-Assisted Laparoscopic Pyeloplasty

Declan G. Murphy, Jamie Kearsley, and Anthony J. Costello

Abstract: Robotic-assisted laparoscopic pyeloplasty (RALP) is an elegant, minimally invasive reconstructive procedure to treat UPJ obstruction. The technique is discussed here in detail. Some selected patients can be discharged within 18 hours. Some series over five years report success rates of between 95 and 100%. The benefits over laparoscopic pyeloplasty are arguable and need to carefully be measured against the increased cost. Perhaps the main advantages are the ease of ureteric spatulation and suturing due to the EndoWrist instruments.

Keywords: Robotic assisted pyeloplasty, UPJ obstruction, Horseshoe kidney

6.1. Introduction

Ureteropelvic junction (UPJ) obstruction is characterized by obstruction to the flow of urine from the renal pelvis to the upper ureter. Hydronephrosis develops as a consequence and progressive renal impairment may ensue if left uncorrected. Primary UPJ obstruction is a congenital condition and is associated with an aberrant crossing vessel to the lower pole in up to 65% of cases (Sampaio 2000). Patients are often

P. Dasgupta (ed.), *Robotic Urological Surgery in Clinical Practice*, 133
DOI: 10.1007/978-1-84800-243-2_6,
© Springer-Verlag London Limited 2008

diagnosed incidentally by ultrasound imaging, though loin pain, hematuria, or urinary tract infection may also be presenting symptoms.

Intravenous urography or isotope diuretic renography are used to confirm the presence of UPJ obstruction. Combining these modalities allows the degree of hydronephrosis, the presence of a high ureteric insertion, the differential function, and the presence of calculi to be ascertained. Contrast CT scanning is useful for detecting aberrant lower pole vessels (see Fig. 6.1).

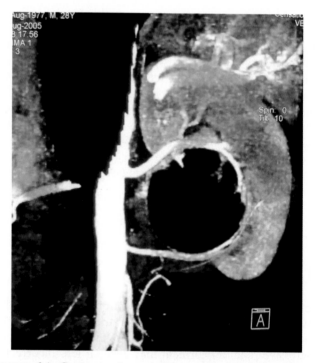

FIGURE 6.1. Contrast-enhanced CT scanning is useful to demonstrate the presence of crossing vessels to the lower pole, a common finding in adult UPJ obstruction.

Progressive loss of renal function or the development of complications such as calculi, are imperative indications for intervention, as is ongoing loin pain.

6.1.1. Management of UPJ Obstruction

A number of minimally invasive techniques have been employed for the management of UPJ obstruction. However, techniques such as antegrade endopyelotomy, retrograde endopyelotomy, and endoscopic balloon dilatation have proved less effective (56–77% success rate) than open pyeloplasty (>90%), which has remained the preferred treatment after many years of experience (Baldwin et al. 2003; O'Reilly et al. 2001; Minervini et al. 2006). In recent years, laparoscopic pyeloplasty has replaced open pyeloplasty in centers where advanced laparoscopic skills are available.

6.1.2. Laparoscopic Pyeloplasty

Laparoscopic pyeloplasty was reported by Schuessler in 1993 (Schuessler et al. 1993). The success rates mirror those of open surgery with 90–95% improvement in clinical and radiologic parameters (Inagaki et al. 2005; Moon et al. 2006). However, dismembered pyeloplasty via the laparoscopic approach remains a challenging procedure for those without considerable laparoscopic experience. Intracorporeal suturing skills are required for reconstruction of the UPJ following resection of the adynamic ureteric segment and reduction of the distended renal pelvis. Even in large series from experienced centers, operating times have remained high, usually due to prolonged anastomotic times (Jarrett et al. 2002). Though no level I or level II evidence exists to justify the superiority of the laparoscopic over the open approach, it appears likely that the benefits to patients of the minimally invasive approach are substantial and that this approach is preferred where available.

6.2. Robotic Technology

The arrival of robotic technology to assist in the performance of complex laparoscopic procedures has had a considerable impact on urologic practice over the past 10 years. Robotic-assisted laparoscopic pyeloplasty (RALP) was first performed in a porcine model using the Zeus^{TM} telerobotic system (Computer Motion, California) (Sung et al. 1999). The Zeus^{TM} was a first-generation "master–slave" system which is no longer commercially available. A group of ten pigs were randomized to either conventional laparoscopic pyeloplasty or RALP using the Zeus^{TM} system. This pilot study concluded that RALP was feasible though no particular advantages were observed with the robotic-assisted approach. Though other reports of RALP using the Zeus^{TM} system have been published (Luke et al. 2004; Lorincz et al. 2005), the surgical robotics market is now dominated by the da Vinci^{TM} surgical system (Intuitive Surgical, California) and the remainder of this chapter relates to the use of this system for RALP.

6.2.1. Advantages and Disadvantages of Robotic Technology

The da Vinci^{TM} surgical system offers a number of technical advances which might be useful in the performance of laparoscopic pyeloplasty. These include:

- Improved depth perception with 3D vision.
- Up to 10x magnification.
- Motion scaling—this allows greater precision when carrying out fine movements.
- Improved degrees-of-freedom using EndoWrist^{TM} technology—this reduces the difficulty associated with complex laparoscopic suturing.
- Articulating EndoWrist^{TM} scissors—this functions as a Potts-type scissors, allowing easy spatulation of the dismembered ureter.

The combined benefit of these features is to reduce the difficulty associated with certain steps of laparoscopic dismembered pyeloplasty.

However, the current generation of robotic technology has a number of disadvantages, including:

- Lack of haptic feedback.
- Bulky robotic arms which may lead to clashing during laparoscopic renal surgery.
- Expensive.

6.3. Technique of RALP

Under general anesthesia and following the administration of prophylactic antibiotics, the patient is placed in the lithotomy position. A cystoscopy is performed and a double-J ureteric stent is placed following a retrograde ureteropyelogram. A urethral catheter is left in the bladder. The patient is then repositioned in a 60° lateral decubitus position with the operating table flexed to its maximum extent (Fig. 6.2). A kidney rest is not routinely used. Care is taken to protect all pressure points.

A four-port transperitoneal approach is used (Fig. 6.3). Pneumoperitoneum is established using a Hasson port in the mid-clavicular line, lateral to the umbilicus. Insufflation pressure is set at 12 mmHg. Two further 8-mm da Vinci^{TM} ports are placed in the iliac fossa and in the hypochondrium, triangulating with the camera port. Though the 12-mm assistant port is often placed laterally during conventional laparoscopic pyeloplasty, the presence of the robotic cart means that this port is more user-friendly when placed in the upper midline (Fig. 6.4)

The 30° down-angle lens is most useful at this stage of the procedure, though the 0° lens may be used later when suturing. The colon is mobilized and the ureter and lower pole of kidney identified. Our preferred instruments at this stage of the procedure are EndoWrist^{TM} bipolar graspers on the left and EndoWrist^{TM} monopolar scissors on the right. The assistant uses a Johannes fenestrated grasper. The UPJ is

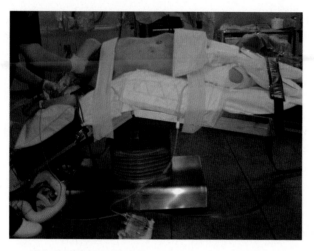

FIGURE 6.2. Patient position for right robotic-assisted laparoscopic pyeloplasty.

fully mobilized and any crossing vessels noted and preserved (Fig. 6.5). The ureter is divided below the UPJ and the renal pelvis is transected and reduced. The adynamic segment is removed. Spatulation of the ureter on its posterior-lateral aspect is accomplished without much difficulty using the angulation on the EndoWrist™ scissors.

We prefer to complete the anterior wall of the anastomosis first rather than the posterior wall. The UPJ is reconstructed (anterior to any crossing vessels) using EndoWrist™ large needle holders as follows.

- A 15-cm 3–0 Vicryl™ stay suture is placed between the apex of the spatulated ureter and the dependent part of the renal pelvis.
- A 20-cm 3–0 Vicryl™ suture is used to complete a running anastomosis along the anterior wall of the reconstructed UPJ. This suture is locked when it reaches the upper limit of the anterior ureteropelvic anastomosis.

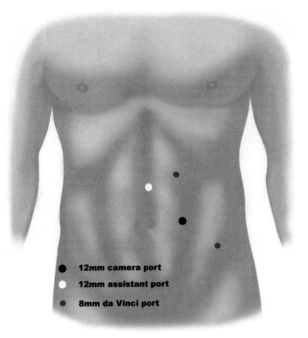

FIGURE 6.3. Port configuration for robotic-assisted left laparoscopic pyeloplasty. A mirror-image configuration is used for right-sided procedures.

- A further 20-cm 3–0 suture is used to close the pyelotomy above the ureteropelvic anastomosis. This running suture is started at the superior aspect of the opened renal pelvis and is secured to the suture which has been locked at the upper end of the anterior anastomotic suture.
- The double-J stent is now replaced in the renal pelvis.
- The posterior edge of the ureteropelvic anastomosis is now closed with a further 3–0 Vicryl™ running suture.

The final appearance demonstrates the reconstructed UPJ anterior to the crossing vessels (Fig. 6.6). A nonsuction tube drain is placed through the lateral 8-mm port and the wounds

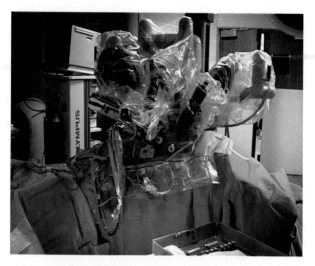

FIGURE 6.4. da Vinci™ cart docked for right robotic-assisted laparoscopic pyeloplasty.

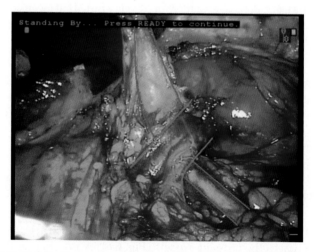

FIGURE 6.5. Aberrant vessels crossing anterior to the left UPJ.

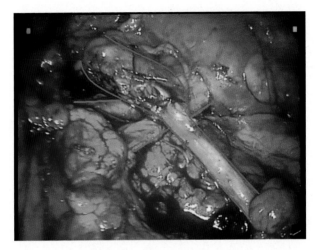

FIGURE 6.6. Appearance post-robotic-assisted laparoscopic left pyeloplasty. The UPJ has been transposed anterior to the crossing vessels.

are closed. Patients are usually discharged within 24 hours and the urethral catheter and drain removed within 3–5 days in the out-patient setting. The double-J stent is removed 6 weeks postoperatively.

6.4. Results of RALP

By the end of 2007, over 200 cases of RALP had been published in the world literature. Some of these series are summarized in Table 6.1.

Gettmann et al. reported their first experience in 2002 following RALP in nine patients (Gettman et al. 2002a). Using a four-port transperitoneal dismembered technique, they reported a mean operating time of 139 (80–215) min, with a mean anastomotic time of 62.4 (40–115) min. One patient required subsequent open surgery to repair a defect

TABLE 6.1. Published series of robotic-assisted laparoscopic pyeloplasty using the da Vinci™ surgical system

Author	N=	Operative time (min)	Suturing time (min)	Complications	Success rate (%)	Follow-up (months)
Bentas	11	197 (110–310)	N/A	None	100	12 (12–27)
Murphy	15	187 (115–240)	47 (27–65)	None	93.3	9 (1–19)
Patel	50	122 (60–330)	22 (10–100)	None	100	11.7 (1–28)
Schwentner	92	108 (72–215)	24.8 (10–115)	5% reoperation rate	96.7	39.1 (3–73)

in the renal pelvis. A 100% success rate was reported but with very limited follow-up (mean of 4.7 months).

Bentas et al. reported their early experience of 11 cases of RALP in 2003 (Bentas et al. 2003). A transperitoneal dismembered technique was used in all cases. They reported a mean operative time of 197 (110–310) min with no intraoperative complications, minimal blood loss, and a 100% success rate at 1 year. It is noteworthy that these authors had no previous experience of laparoscopic pyeloplasty.

We published our own experience of 15 RALP when reporting our overall experience with robotic-assisted laparoscopic renal surgery (Murphy et al. 2008). This group included six pediatric and nine adult patients. The mean operative time was 187 (115–240) min with a mean suturing time of 47 (27–65) min. We noted in particular that the suturing time reduced considerably over the most recent five cases, averaging less than 30 min. One patient was lost to followup but the remaining 14 patients had excellent clinical and radiologic outcomes at a mean follow-up of 9 (1–19) months. Our series also featured three patients who were discharged within 18 hours of RALP, highlighting the minimally invasive nature of this procedure.

Patel et al. reported the outcomes of 50 dismembered RALP (Patel 2005). The operative time averaged 122 (60–330) min with a mean anastomotic time of only 20 (10–100) min. There were no reported complications. At a mean follow-up of 11.7 (1–28) months all 50 patients were doing well clinically and radiologically.

The largest reported series at this time is that of Schwentner et al. (Schwentner et al. 2007). This group updated the results of Gettmann (Gettman et al. 2002a) and others (Peschel et al. 2004) who had reported the early RALP results from Innsbruck. With a mean follow-up of 39.1 (3–73) months, they reported their series of 92 patients who had undergone dismembered RALP over a 5-year period. Crossing vessels were noted in 45 patients. The mean operating time was 108 (72–215) min though this had reduced considerably as their experience developed. The last 12 cases had a mean operating time of 89 (72–112) min. The overall mean anastomotic time was 24.8 (10–115) min. An antegrade approach was used to place the double-J stent intraoperatively in 87 patients. Malposition of the stent led to ureteroscopy in three patients. Three other patients required early operative reintervention. This included two patients who hemorrhaged into the collecting system, one of which required percutaneous nephrostomy and stent exchange and one of which required redo-open pyeloplasty at 3 months. The third patient had a urine leak and required open exploration to close a large defect in the renal pelvis. The overall success rate was 96.7%.

6.4.1. Conventional vs. Robotic-Assisted Laparoscopic Pyeloplasty

Conflicting conclusions are drawn from two studies which have sought to compare RALP with standard laparoscopic pyeloplasty. In a nonrandomized comparison, Gettman's group reported shorter operative and anastomotic times with RALP compared to pure laparoscopic pyeloplasty (Gettman et al. 2002b). The total operative and suturing times were 140 and 70 min compared to 235 and 120 min for robotic and laparoscopic pyeloplasty, respectively. However, Kavoussi's group have reported longer operating times and significantly higher costs associated with the robotic approach in a small comparative trial ($n = 20$) (Link et al. 2006). Operative costs were 2.7-times higher in the robotic group (1.7-times if the capital costs were excluded). There are no randomized trials to compare the conventional and robotic-assisted laparoscopic approaches.

6.4.2. RALP in Special Situations

Two of the more challenging situations when considering pyeloplasty are the presence of a horseshoe kidney, and previous failed treatment of UPJ obstruction (secondary

UPJ obstruction). RALP has been reported for both situations. Chammas et al. reported their RALP experience with three horseshoe kidneys using the da Vinci™ surgical system (Chammas et al. 2006). A transperitoneal 4-port approach was used. The isthmus was not divided. The mean operating time was 148 (125–170) min with minimal blood loss. The only reported complication was an episode of pyelonephritis which responded well to antibiotics. With a mean follow-up of 21 (13–29) months, all three patients had good clinical and radiologic outcomes.

The series from Innsbruck includes two patients with horseshoe kidneys (Schwentner et al. 2007). The isthmus was divided in both cases using monopolar cautery, sutures, and a bolster as necessary. The lower pole on each side was nephropexed to the psoas to ensure a straight reconstructed UPJ with no kinking. Both patients had an uneventful recovery with good outcomes.

Our own experience at Guy's includes dismembered pyeloplasties for two horseshoe kidneys. The isthmus was not divided in either case. Operative time averaged 170 min with no significant complications. Both patients had satisfactory outcomes. There is frequently complex vascular anatomy in these cases, often with branches from the common iliac artery. We adjust our port positions to have the camera port at the umbilicus and the remaining ports placed more caudal than described above.

Secondary UPJ obstruction presents a challenging situation. Schwentner's large series of 92 patients includes 12 who had previous intervention for UPJ obstruction (Schwentner et al. 2007). Of these, three had undergone previous nondismembered pyeloplasty and nine had undergone endopyelotomy. One of these 12 patients required early open reoperation to close a defect in the renal pelvis and subsequently made a good recovery with no long-term sequelae. The remaining 11 patients underwent uncomplicated RALP with a good outcome.

Patel's series of 50 patients included five who had undergone previous intervention for UPJ obstruction (Patel 2005).

Of these, three had undergone pyeloplasty and two had undergone endopyelotomy. No complications were reported for this sub-group and they form part of a series with a 100% overall success rate.

6.5. Conclusions

It is apparent that the da Vinci™ surgical system is a useful tool for laparoscopic dismembered pyeloplasty. The additional degrees-of-freedom are not only useful for the reconstructive aspect of this procedure, but also for the mobilization of the renal pelvis especially when crossing vessels are present. The additional angulation provided by the robotic instruments facilitates prompt progression throughout the dissection. The benefits of wristed instruments for laparoscopic suturing are well recognized and are particularly useful when complex reconstruction is required such as in dismembered pyeloplasty.

The available data suggests that RALP is feasible and safe, and produces clinical outcomes comparable to those of laparoscopic and open pyeloplasty. There is clearly a health economic issue regarding the funding of this expensive technology, but the likely reduction in learning curve for surgeons, and in recuperation time for patients, may help offset the investment. Further developments in the field of surgical robotics will hopefully lead to more affordable, less bulky equipment with the addition of haptic feedback to mimic tactile sensation.

References

Baldwin DD, Dunbar JA, Wells N, McDougall EM (2003) Single-center comparison of laparoscopic pyeloplasty, Acucise endopyelotomy, and open pyeloplasty. J Endourol 17(3):155–160

Bentas W, Wolfram M, Brautigam R, Probst M, Beecken WD, Jonas D et al. (2003) Da Vinci robot assisted Anderson-Hynes dismembered pyeloplasty: technique and 1 year follow-up. World J Urol 21(3):133–138

Chammas M, Jr., Feuillu B, Coissard A, Hubert J (2006) Laparoscopic robotic-assisted management of pelvi-ureteric junction obstruction in patients with horseshoe kidneys: technique and 1-year follow-up. BJU Int 97(3):579–583

Gettman MT, Neururer R, Bartsch G, Peschel R (2002a) Anderson-Hynes dismembered pyeloplasty performed using the da Vinci robotic system. Urology 60(3):509–513

Gettman MT, Peschel R, Neururer R, Bartsch G (2002b) A comparison of laparoscopic pyeloplasty performed with the daVinci robotic system versus standard laparoscopic techniques: initial clinical results. Eur Urol 42(5):453–457

Inagaki T, Rha KH, Ong AM, Kavoussi LR, Jarrett TW (2005) Laparoscopic pyeloplasty: current status. BJU Int 95 Suppl 2: 102–105

Jarrett TW, Chan DY, Charambura TC, Fugita O, Kavoussi LR (2002) Laparoscopic pyeloplasty: the first 100 cases. J Urol 167(3):1253–1256

Link RE, Bhayani SB, Kavoussi LR (2006) A prospective comparison of robotic and laparoscopic pyeloplasty. Ann Surg 243(4):486–491

Lorincz A, Knight CG, Kant AJ, Langenburg SE, Rabah R, Gidell K et al. (2005) Totally minimally invasive robot-assisted unstented pyeloplasty using the Zeus Microwrist Surgical System: an animal study. J Pediatr Surg 40(2):418–422

Luke PP, Girvan AR, Al OM, Beasley KA, Carson M (2004) Laparoscopic robotic pyeloplasty using the Zeus Telesurgical System. Can J Urol 11(5):2396–2400

Minervini A, Davenport K, Keeley FX Jr, Timoney AG (2006) Antegrade versus retrograde endopyelotomy for pelvi-ureteric junction (PUJ) obstruction. Eur Urol 49(3):536–542

Moon DA, El-Shazly MA, Chang CM, Gianduzzo TR, Eden CG (2006) Laparoscopic pyeloplasty: evolution of a new gold standard. Urology 67(5):932–936

Murphy DG, Challacombe BJ, Olsburgh J et al. (2008) Ablative and reconstructive robotic-assisted laparoscopic renal surgery. Int J Clin Pract. 2008 Feb 9. [Epub ahead of Print]

O'Reilly PH, Brooman PJ, Mak S, Jones M, Pickup C, Atkinson C et al. (2001) The long-term results of Anderson-Hynes pyeloplasty. BJU Int 87(4):287–289

148   D.G. Murphy et al.

Patel V (2005) Robotic-assisted laparoscopic dismembered pyelo-
plasty. Urology 66(1):45–49
Peschel R, Neururer R, Bartsch G, Gettman MT (2004) Robotic
pyeloplasty: technique and results. Urol Clin North Am
31(4):737–741
Sampaio FJ (2000) Renal anatomy. Endourologic considerations.
Urol Clin North Am 27(4):585–607, vii
Schuessler WW, Grune MT, Tecuanhuey LV, Preminger GM (1993)
Laparoscopic dismembered pyeloplasty. J Urol 150(6):1795–1799
Sung GT, Gill IS, Hsu TH (1999) Robotic-assisted laparoscopic
pyeloplasty: a pilot study. Urology : 53(6):1099–1103
Schwentner C, Pelzer A, Neururer R, Springer B, Horninger W,
Bartsch G et al. (2007) Robotic Anderson-Hynes pyeloplasty:
5-year experience of one centre. BJU Int 100(4):880–885

Chapter 7
Robotic Pediatric Urology

Iqbal S. Shergill, Manit Arya, and Imran Mushtaq

Abstract: With the widespread uptake of robotic surgery in the field of adult urology, attention has recently shifted to applying this technology to conditions in the pediatric population. The requirement for minimally invasive treatments and the reconstructive nature of pediatric urologic surgery makes robotic technology very appealing in this specialty. This chapter describes the current uses and recent advances of robotics in pediatric urology.

Keywords: Paediatric, Pyeloplasty, Heminephrectomy, Ureteric reimplantation

7.1. Introduction

There is no doubt that the use of robotic technology in pediatric urology is very much in its infancy. Although many of the same principles from the adult population can be applied, several technical details vary in the pediatric population. The benefits of using the robot, such as greater ability to perform precise suturing, enhanced stereoscopic visualization offering true depth-of-field vision (Fig. 7.1), with improvements in difficult dissection, and increased dexterity, must clearly outweigh the inherent disadvantages, which include increased cost, lack of tactile feedback, and the current lack of pediatric sized ports and instruments. Although many of the same principles from the adult population can be applied, the main

P. Dasgupta (ed.), *Robotic Urological Surgery in Clinical Practice*,   149
DOI: 10.1007/978-1-84800-243-2_7,
© Springer-Verlag London Limited 2008

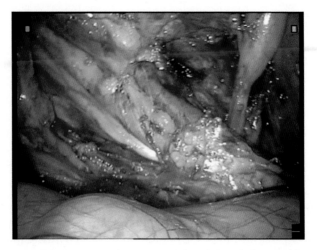

FIGURE 7.1. Retrocaval ureter on the right of the photograph clearly shown to be traversing behind the inferior vena cava.

technical difference in the pediatric population is the placement of the ports, which is a cornerstone in robotic surgery in children. The limited retroperitoneal space of infants means that the depth of insertion of the ports and instruments has to be kept to a minimum, otherwise the extracorporeal movement of the instrument arms increases, resulting in collisions between the arms (this is partly overcome by more extensive use of the wrist movements). On the basis of the above factors, one would naturally assume that the surgical management of both upper and lower tract pathologies would benefit from the use of the robot. In particular, it would be expected that reconstructive surgery would particularly benefit. The uptake of robotic surgery in pediatric urology has been slow and limited to major centers only. The current uses and relevant clinical studies are reviewed.

7.2. Pyeloplasty

Open pyeloplasty in children is traditionally performed through the retroperitoneal approach as this has several potential advantages with regard to urine leakage and avoidance of injury to intra-abdominal organs. On the basis of these principles and the original concept of retroperitoneal laparoscopic pyeloplasty in children (Yeung et al. 2001), Olsen et al. published the first report on robotic-assisted retroperitoneoscopic pyeloplasty (Olsen and Jorgensen 2004). In this study on 13 children, 15 pyeloplasties were performed using the da Vinci^{TM} surgical system. The procedures were completed in all cases, with a median operative time of 173 min (range 76 to 215) and there were no perioperative complications. Median postoperative hospital stay was 2 days (range 1 to 3) and only two patients had postoperative complications, which were related to the double-J stent (one patient had displacement of the stent with its lower end in the distal ureter, and the other patient was rehospitalized with occlusion of the stent). In their follow-up period, all patients had a satisfactory outcome. Interestingly, they concluded that robotic-assisted retroperitoneal pyeloplasty in children was feasible with shorter operative time and similar complications as in standard retroperitoneoscopic procedures. Since that initial report, no further publications on retroperitoneal access with the robotic system have been published until the same group reported their 5-year experience (Olsen et al. 2007). In this study, a total of 65 children (median age 7.9 years, range 1.7 to 17.1) underwent 67 pyeloplasties over a four-year period. Median operative time was 143 min (range 93 to 300) and complications occurred in 12 of the 67 procedures. The complications were urinary tract infection, transient hematuria, displaced ureteric catheter, and the need for postoperative temporary nephrostomy. One case was converted to open surgery due to lack of space and limitations in the movement of the camera arm. Longer-term complications included repeat surgery due to a kinking ureter, an overlooked aberrant vessel, and decreasing differential function on renography necessitating balloon dilatation. In the other 55 procedures follow-up was uneventful. They concluded that robotic-assisted retroperitoneoscopic pyeloplasty gave more direct access to the ureteropelvic junction, allowed shorter operative times with results and complication rates comparable to transperitoneal robotic-assisted pyeloplasty, as well as laparoscopic and open pyeloplasty in children.

The transperitoneal approach in children has recently been compared to open pyeloplasty in two series (Lee et al. 2006; Yee et al. 2006). Lee et al. (2006) compared 33 age-matched children undergoing open and robotic-assisted laparoscopic pyeloplasty for safety, efficacy, operative time, blood loss, in-hospital narcotic use, and length of stay. Robotic pyeloplasty was deemed safe and efficacious with advantages of decreased hospital stay, decreased narcotic use, and operative times approaching those of open surgery. In the other study, Yee et al. (2006) compared the initial results of the da Vinci™ robotic-assisted laparoscopic pyeloplasty versus open Anderson–Hynes pyeloplasty in eight children matched by age group [mean age was 11.5 years (range 6.4 to 16.5) in the robotic-assisted group and 9.8 years (range 6.0 to 15.6) in the open group]. They found that although robotic-assisted laparoscopic pyeloplasty appeared to decrease the length of hospitalization and use of pain medication, it was associated with a longer mean operative time (363 min in the robotic-assisted group versus 248 min in the open group). Most recently, Kutikov et al. (2006) reported on their experience of robotic-assisted pyeloplasty, with a mean operative duration of 122.8 min in infants (mean age 5.6 months). In this small series of nine patients, seven were reported to have resolution or improvement in hydronephrosis and two had no evidence of obstruction on follow-up diuretic renography.

It appears that initial studies have shown that robotic-assisted pyeloplasty is technically feasible and safe, with operative times now approaching that of the standard open procedure and suturing in dismembered pyeloplasty with the robot being straightforward. Whether this translates into any significant overall advantage as compared with the current standard of care is debatable, and the costs of obtaining and maintaining the robot also need to be taken into consideration. Additional clinical experience is required to determine the long-term efficacy of robotic pyeloplasty, and as robotic technology improves, it is anticipated that this method of repair may become the minimally invasive treatment of choice.

7.3. Heminephrectomy

Duplex anomalies and the complications associated with them are commonly seen in pediatric urologic practice. The role of the robot in the management of heminephrectomy (partial nephrectomy) seems to be appealing, theoretically allowing careful dissection and reconstruction during surgery, however, published clinical experience has been rather limited. One of the first reports was by Pedraza et al. (2004b) who performed bilateral robotic-assisted laparoscopic heminephroureterectomy, in a 4-year-old girl. They used the da Vinci™ robot to dissect the renal hilum and upper pole vessels, and isolate the upper pole segment. The upper pole segment was then excised using a Harmonic scalpel and an argon beam coagulator was used to fulgurate the base of the upper pole segment. The patient was then repositioned and a similar procedure was performed on the right side. They reported no intraoperative or postoperative complications, an overall surgical time of 7 hours and 20 min and an estimated blood loss of only 15 ml. The patient required only simple analgesia postoperatively and two doses of supplemental narcotic analgesia. She was discharged home on the second postoperative day and returned to full activity in 2 weeks. Subsequently, Olsen et al. (2005) investigated the feasibility of performing robotic-assisted upper pole heminephrectomy in 14 girls using the retroperitoneal approach with the da Vinci™ system. The upper pole was removed by diathermy or ultrasonic scissors (which did not have the option of wrist movement of the normal robotic instruments). Their median operative time was 176 min (range 120–360 min) and in two cases, open operation had to be performed due to lack of progress and bleeding. They concluded that although there were several advantages in using the robot in the retroperitoneum, further development of the instruments was required before the resection of a nonfunctioning upper pole could be firmly included in the spectrum of indications. Current evidence suggests that robotic-assisted heminephrectomy may be of clinical benefit, but certain refinements, especially with instrumentation, have to be made before its use can be fully assessed for this purpose. Quite clearly long-term results and comparisons with open and laparoscopic techniques are awaited.

7.4. Pelvic Surgery

Minimally invasive laparoscopic and robotic procedures have been shown to have significant advantages in pelvic surgery in adults as compared to the open approach. The excellent visualization and three-dimensional movements potentially allow the ability to perform delicate manipulations behind the bladder with control and confidence. Almost a decade ago, descriptions of laparoscopic antireflux surgery were reported, but never achieved popularity predominantly due to the difficulty in dissection and suturing. The advantages of the robot have now allowed the reintroduction of pelvic surgery in children including careful suturing of the bladder, urethra, and ureters.

Olsen et al. (2003) reported the success of the transvesical robotic-assisted approach for transtrigonal Cohen ureteric reimplantation in an animal model. More recently, both extra- and intravesical robotic-assisted approaches for antireflux surgery in children have been reported (Peters and Woo 2005). This is only possible with appropriate instruments, which allow the pediatric urologist the maneuverability during the development of the submucosal tunnel and the suturing of the vesicoureteral anastomosis. The robotic-assisted Lich–Gregoir procedure has been documented (Peters 2004), although the authors have not definitively recommended this technique in routine practice. This is because reflux was persistent in two out of 17 patients, suggesting that robotic surgery may not provide an adequate tunnel. In comparison, the success rate of open extravesical ureteroplasty is generally considered to be nearly 100%. Additionally, in using a robotic technique in very young children with small bladder capacities, there are worries regarding adequate closure of the bladder because the current working instruments of the da Vinci™ system are 8 mm and the camera port is 12 mm. However, the introduction of the smaller 5-mm instruments should prove to be more advantageous and efficacious.

7.5. Other Procedures

It is only inevitable, that a wider range of surgical procedures will be performed with the aid of the robot in the pediatric urologic population, based on improved surgical technique, confidence, experience, and creativity. Technically complex procedures such as Mitrofanoff channel (Pedraza et al. 2004a) and the surgical management of retrocaval ureter (Gundeti et al. 2006) have been successfully performed with the aid of the robot (Fig. 7.2). More recently, Lee et al. have demonstrated the feasibility of robotic-assisted pyelolithotomy in complex stone cases (Lee et al. 2007). As is well known, patients with cystinuria require multiple surgical procedures throughout their lifetime, and hence the least invasive, safest,

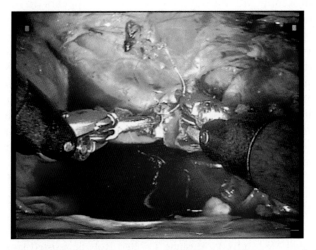

FIGURE 7.2. Dismembered retrocaval ureter being precisely sutured robotically anterior to the inferior vena cava.

and most efficient approach should be used to render them stone-free. Lee et al. (2007) retrospectively reviewed their experience with robotic pyelolithotomy in five patients, with a mean age at surgery of 16.6 years, and mean follow-up of 15.4 months. They found this procedure to be safe and efficacious. Mean operative time was 315.4 (normal text) min (range 165.0 to 462.0), and mean estimated blood loss was 19.0 ml (0.0 to 50.0). Mean hospital stay was 3.8 days (range 2.3 to 5.7), and mean narcotic usage was 2.1 mg/kg morphine (1.5 to 3.5). Of the four cases completed robotically three were rendered stone-free and one had a residual 6-mm lower pole stone. One patient with a cystine staghorn calculus required conversion to an open procedure because of inability to remove the stone.

7.6. Conclusions

Robotic technology in pediatric urologic surgery is currently in its infancy. Overall, the early results with robotic-assisted laparoscopy are encouraging and there appears to be a rapidly growing body of evidence to support that this type of surgery is technically possible, safe, and efficacious. The reconstructive nature of pediatric urology lends itself to the advantages of robotic technology. In particular, pyeloplasty, heminephrectomy, lower tract ureteric reimplantation, and antireflux surgery may be best served with this technology. Building on the experience gained in the adult population, various procedures may be adapted to suit the pediatric patient. Further evidence, in the form of prospective trials should be encouraged and supported to meet this end.

References

Gundeti MS, Duffy P, Mushtaq I (2006) Robotic-assisted laparoscopic correction of pediatric retrocaval ureter. J Laparoendosc Adv Surg Tech A 16(4):422–424

Kutikov A, Nguyen M, Guzzo T, Canter D, Casale P (2006) Robot assisted pyeloplasty in the infant-lessons learned. J Urol 176(5):2237–2239

Lee RS, Retik AB, Borer JG, Peters CA (2006) Pediatric robot assisted laparoscopic dismembered pyeloplasty: comparison with a cohort of open surgery. J Urol 175:683

Lee RS, Passerotti CC, Estrada CR, Borer JG, Peters CA (2007) Early Results of Robot Assisted Laparoscopic Lithotomy in Adolescents. J Urol 177:2306–2310

Olsen LH, Deding D, Yeung CK, Jorgensen TM (2003) Computer assisted laparoscopic pneumovesical ureter reimplantation a.m. Cohen: initial experience in a pig model. APMIS Suppl 109:23–25

Olsen LH, Jorgensen TM (2004) Computer assisted pyeloplasty in children: the retroperitoneal approach. J Urol 171:2629

Olsen LH, Jørgensen TM (2005) Robotically assisted retroperitoneoscopic heminephrectomy in children: initial clinical results. J Pediatr Urol 1:101e4

Olsen L, Rawashdeh Y, Jorgensen T (2007) Pediatric robot assisted retroperitoneoscopic pyeloplasty: a 5-year experience. J Urol 178(5):2137–2141

Pedraza R, Weiser A, Franco I (2004a) Laparoscopic appendicovesicostomy (Mitrofanoff procedure) in a child using the da Vinci robotic system. Urol 171(4):1652–1653

Pedraza R, Palmer L, Moss V, Franco I (2004b) Bilateral robotic assisted laparoscopic hemi-nephroureterectomy. J Urol 171:2394–2395

Peters CA (2004) Robotically assisted surgery in pediatric urology. Urol Clin North Am 31:743e52

Peters CA, Woo R (2005) Intravesical robotically assisted bilateral ureteral reimplantation. J Endourol 19:618–622

Yee DS, Shanberg AM, Duel BP, Rodriguez E, Eichel L, Rajpoot D (2006) Initial comparison of robotic-assisted laparoscopic versus open pyeloplasty in children. Urology 67:599

Yeung CK, Tam YH, Sihoe JD, Lee KH, Liu KW (2001) Retroperitoneoscopic dismembered pyeloplasty for pelvi-ureteric junction obstruction in infants and children. BJU Int 87:509

Chapter 8
Robotic Gynecology/Urogynecology

Kankipati Shanti Raju, Andreas John Papadopoulos, and Mohammad Shamim Khan

Abstract: Robotic hysterectomy is the commonest gynaeco-logical procedure and has the potential of becoming as impor-tant as robotic radical prostatectomy. Myomectomy is another important application of robotic surgery. In pelvic reconstruc-tion, robotics has a particular role in sacro-colpopexy and vesico-vaginal fistula repair where non-randomised results are as good as open and laparoscopic surgery. A few cases of robotic colposuspension have been reported.

Keywords: robotics, hysterectomy, myomectomy, sacro-colpopexy, colposuspension

8.1. Introduction

There has been an increasing demand for minimally invasive surgery in all surgical disciplines. Gynecology and urogyne-cology are no exceptions. Laparoscopic surgery has served as a very useful diagnostic and therapeutic tool in the man-agement of a broad spectrum of gynecologic conditions. It is claimed that almost all types of gynecologic procedures can be performed through a laparoscope (Nezhat et al. 2000). Universal application of laparoscopy in these surgical specialties has however, been hampered by a number of

P. Dasgupta (ed.), *Robotic Urological Surgery in Clinical Practice*, 159
DOI: 10.1007/978-1-84800-243-2_8,
© Springer-Verlag London Limited 2008

limitations of standard laparoscopic technology. These include a long learning curve, two-dimensional visualization, and counter-intuitive motion due to the fulcrum effect offering the surgeon only four degrees-of-freedom of movement. The restricted movement of instruments within the abdomen and pelvis poses significant difficulty during operations in this confined space. Moreover laparoscopy is not ergonomically friendly and difficulties are compounded by hand tremors (Styolopoulos and Rattner 2003).

Robotic technology represents a technological advance in the evolution of minimally invasive surgery. Current robotic surgical systems have resulted in a paradigm shift in the minimally invasive approach to complex surgical procedures. In addition to movements of the robotic instruments being intuitive, it also provides the surgeon with seven degrees-of-freedom, 540° of wristing, motion scaling, tremor elimination, and ease of suturing with both hands in the restricted area of the pelvis. The surgeon is comfortably seated at a console, remote from the patient and benefits from the 3-D stereoscopic vision with 10x magnification; this makes surgery more ergonomic and precise. Robotic-assisted surgery is gaining ever increasing popularity as its inherent advantages allow the surgeons to overcome obstacles encountered in conventional laparoscopic procedures. Whereas urologists have been at the forefront of grasping this cutting-edge technology to perform complex pelvic surgical procedures, their gynecology and urogynecology colleagues have been relatively slow in embracing this. However, this trend seems to be changing.

This chapter will examine the recent experience of robotic-assisted technology in the field of gynecologic and urogynecologic surgery and discuss its possible future applications to this field.

8.2. Robotic Gynecologic Surgery

Over the past 5 years robotic-assisted surgery has been evaluated to various degrees in gynecology. In 1999 Falcone et al. described tubal anastomosis using robotic-assisted techniques. In 2002 Diaz-Arrastia et al. used computer-enhanced robotic surgery to perform laparoscopic hysterectomy in 11 patients. In 2004 Advincula et al. reported laparoscopic myomectomy with robotic assistance in 31 patients. Table 8.1 illustrates the gynecologic surgical procedures performed by robotic-assisted surgery.

8.3. Theatre Setup

In robotic-assisted gynecologic surgery patients are placed in a dorsal lithotomy position using stirrups as for conventional laparoscopic procedures. Bowel preparation is used according to the surgeon's preference with a view to decompress the distal bowel for improved pelvic visualization (Advincula 2006). The bladder is emptied at the start of the procedure or a catheter left in situ. Depending on the procedure being performed a uterine manipulator may be used with or without a Koch colpotomy ring and vaginal pneumo-occluder balloon (Cooper Surgical, Trumbull, CT). Four trocars are usually placed (see Fig. 8.1); a 12-mm transumbilical, two low lateral 5-mm ports, and an accessory 10-mm port. Investigators have recommended starting the surgery with a standard laparoscope and then switching to robotic-assisted surgery but it is likely that with more experience this two-stage approach could be abandoned (Nezhat et al. 2006). The lateral 5-mm ports are exchanged for 8-mm robotic ports when the robot is to be used. These 8-mm ports are mounted onto the two operating arms of the da Vinci™ system. The patient is placed in a steep Trendelenburg position once all the desired ports are in place. The surgical cart is then positioned in the middle next to the patient's legs or between the legs depending on the procedure to be performed and the robot is docked. Each port is thus attached to a robotic arm with the exception of the accessory ports. The surgical assistant at the bedside exchanges the EndoWrist instruments and deals with the accessory port. Nezhat et al. (2006) have reported a mean assembly time of 18.9 min, the time to switch from laparoscope to robot (moving the robot,

TABLE 8.1 Gynecologic surgical procedures suited to robotic-assisted surgery

Hysterectomy	AAGS type IIB	Laparoscopic assisted vaginal hysterectomy—cardinal and uterosacral ligaments secured vaginally
	AAGS type III	Laparoscopic supracervical hysterectomy
	AAGS type IVE	Total laparoscopic removal of uterus and cervix, with vault closure
Myomectomy		
Tubal reanastomosis		
Ovarian transposition		
Ovarian cysts	Ovarian cyst	Ovarian cystectomy
	Oophorectomy	
Endometriosis	Ovarian cyst	
	Rectovaginal and pelvic lesions	
Urogynecology	Bladder neck suspension procedures	
	Sacrocolpopexy	

TABLE 8.1 Continued

Gyne-oncology	Endometrial endometrioid cancer	Surgical staging: hysterectomy, bilateral salpingo-oophorectomy with lymphadenectomy
	Endometrial serous cancer	As above + omentectomy +/-paraortic LND
	Cervical cancer	Radical hysterectomy with pelvic and para-aortic lymph nodes
	Ovarian cancer	Staging, interval debulking, omentectomy, hysterectomy and BSO and LND (pelvic + para-aortic), bowel resection
	Central pelvic recurrence of gynecologic tumors	Exenteration (anterior, posterior, total)
Genetic carriers of gene defects	BRCA1, BRCA2 carriers	Prophylactic salpingo-oophorectomy

For American Association of Gynecologic Laparoscopists Classification (AAGL) please see Table 8.2

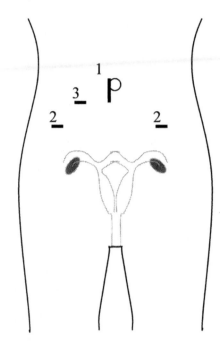

FIGURE 8.1 Port placement (3–4 armed system) for gynecologic procedures. *1*) 12-mm transumbilical port, *2*) two lower lateral 8-mm ports, *3*) 5–15 mm accessory to right and/or left and lateral to umbilicus

changing the 5 to 8-mm ports, changing camera, and surgical instrument allowing the surgeon to operate from the console). The mean disassembly time was reported as 2.1 min to switch from robot to laparoscopy to close the sites (moving the robot, changing camera, and surgical instruments to allow the surgeon to finish).

8.4. Hysterectomy

Hysterectomy has been the main surgical procedure performed by gynecologists throughout the latter part of the last century. This procedure has undergone significant evolutionary changes as a result of the advent of minimally invasive surgical techniques. This evolution is marked by transformation from abdominal and vaginal hysterectomy, through the laparoscopic-assisted vaginal approach (Raju and Auld 1994), to laparoscopic subtotal and finally total laparoscopic hysterectomy. The use of the robotic platform allows the principles of open surgery to be followed. The vascular pedicles can be secured with prior dissection using sutures or radiofrequency current. The American Association of Gynecologic Laparoscopists (AAGL), have classified laparoscopic hysterectomy into different types as depicted in Table 8.2.

TABLE 8.2 Classification system for laparoscopic hysterectomy from Olive et al. (2000)

Type 0	Laparoscopic-directed preparation for vaginal hysterectomy
Type I	Dissection up to but excluding uterine arteries
	IA Dissection up to but excluding uterine arteries
	IB IA with anterior structures
	IC IA with posterior culdotomy
	ID IA with anterior structures and posterior culdotomy
Type II	Type I with occlusion and division of uterine arteries (unilateral/bilateral)
	IIA Type I with occlusion + division of uterine arteries
	IIB–IID as above
Type III	Type II with part of cardinal-uterosacral ligament complex only (unilateral/bilateral)
	IIIA Type II with part of cardinal-uterosacral ligament complex only
	IIIB–IIID as above
Type IV	Type II with complete cardinal-uterosacral ligament complex only (unilateral/bilateral)
	IVA Type II with complete cardinal-uterosacral ligament complex only
	IVB–IVD as above
	IVE Laparoscopically directed removal of entire uterus

In the series reported by Diaz-Arrastia et al. (2002) the hysterectomy performed was AAGL-type IIB. The procedure was performed as a laparoscopic-assisted vaginal hysterectomy with the cardinal and uterosacral ligaments being secured vaginally. Eleven patients underwent surgery with an operating time between 270 and 600 min. One patient required open conversion and the average hospital stay was 2 days. In contrast Beste et al. (2005) performed AAGL-type IVE hysterectomy using the da Vinci system in 11 patients. The entire procedure in type-IVE hysterectomy is performed laparoscopically including removal of the uterus with cervix and vaginal vault closure. The operating time was short ranging from 148 to 277 min.

Reynolds and Advincula (2006) performed both IVE hysterectomy and LSH III (laparoscopic supra-cervical hysterectomy) in 16 patients with no open conversion. Operating time varied from 170 to 432 min, with a hospital stay of 1.5 days. Fiorentino et al. (2006) reported 18 patients who underwent type-IVE hysterectomy, two requiring open conversion because of poor visualization.

The largest series of total laparoscopic hysterectomy (IVE) was published by Kho et al. (2007). Their series of 91 patients also included hysterectomies with and without appendicectomy and lysis of adhesions. They noted that operative time reduced with experience. A single intraoperative complication was a small bowel tear which was repaired using robotic assistance in a patient with extensive adhesions.

Some authors have reported that presence of adhesions is not a contraindication to robotic operations. It is possible to divide the adhesions and this is quoted as an additional advantage of robotic assistance (Advincula and Reynolds 2005; Reynolds and Advincula 2006). Clearly, a direct comparison with laparoscopic total hysterectomy needs to be made in a clinical trial setting.

8.5. Reproductive Surgery

8.5.1. Myomectomy

Current management of leiomyomata must take into consideration the future fertility requirements of the patient (Kenney and Papadopoulos 2001). The most frequent option for women who wish to retain fertility is myomectomy either transabdominal or transvaginal hysteroscopic resection. Several studies including two prospective trials have demonstrated that laparoscopic management reduces operative morbidity and time to recovery (Mais et al. 1996; Seracchioli et al. 2000). However, the open transabdominal excision is still the most commonly practiced procedure for sub-serous and intramural fibroids. This is possibly a reflection of the advanced surgical skills required for enucleation and multilayer closure of the defect. In addition the risk of uterine rupture during subsequent pregnancy and higher risk of recurrence (Doridot et al. 2001) may impede the use of minimally invasive techniques to treat these conditions.

Senapati and Advincula (2007) have reported myomectomy using the da Vinci system and described how they overcame the complexities of the procedure encountered during conventional laparoscopy. MRI (magnetic resonance imaging) staging is recommended prior to surgery to exclude adenomyosis and also to determine the exact location and size of the myomas, to allow precision in hysterotomy incision. Vasopressin is used intraoperatively to reduce bleeding into the operating field. Usually the uterine incision for the myomectomy with conventional laparoscopic surgery is made transversely as this aids closure with rigid instruments. In open myomectomy incision can be made in any position usually longitudinally and this is also possible with the robotic system. The fibroid is removed with a tissue morcellator as with conventional laparoscopy. It has been noted in conventional laparoscopic fibroid removal that the combination of a pneumoperitoneum, vasopressin, and ability to see magnified dissection planes allows reduced blood loss compared to open myomectomy. These advantages are also seen with difficult fibroid removal using robotic-assisted surgery.

The largest published series of myomectomy consists of 35 cases from Advincula et al. (2004). The mean diameter was 7.9 ± 3.5 cm (95% CI 6.6–9.1), for a mean myoma count of 1.6 (range 1–5). No blood transfusions were required for a mean blood loss of 169 ± 198.7 ml (95% CI 99.1–238.4). The average length of surgery was 230.8 ± 83 min (95% CI 201.6–260), and the median length of stay was 1 day although others have stated that the procedure can be performed on an outpatient basis (Advincula and Song 2007). In this series from Advincula et al. (2004) three cases required open conversion; in two cases lack of haptic (tactile) feedback made leiomyoma enucleation difficult whereas in the third case vasopressin-induced cardiogenic shock necessitated conversion. It was noted that robotic assistance improved maneuverability with the instrumentation improving dissection from a variety of angles. The seated surgeon can repair the hysterotomy in a multi-layer fashion using the robot assistance similar to the open procedure.

8.5.2. Tubal Anastomosis

A few papers have been published using the modern robotic platforms for microsurgery involving tubal anastomosis (Degueldre et al. 2000, Cadiere et al. 2001). These authors describe an average operating time of 50 min per tube which was not significantly different from open microsurgery (Degueldre et al. 2000). However, the lack of haptic or tactile feedback was noted as a major disadvantage.

8.5.3. Ovarian Transposition

Ovarian transposition is often required in premenopausal women requiring pelvic radiotherapy for malignant conditions in order to conserve ovarian function. This procedure involves the repositioning of the ovaries outside the pelvis into the abdomen. This procedure can be performed laparoscopically and has been the subject of numerous publications (Bisharah and Tulandi 2003). In 2003 Molpus et al. (2003) described a case using robotic-assisted techniques in a patient with stage-IB1 cervical squamous cancer prior to radiotherapy. Preserved ovarian function was noted following radiotherapy treatment with normal levels of follicle stimulating and luteinizing hormone.

8.6. Endometriosis

Minimally invasive techniques have been extensively utilized in the diagnosis, and treatment of endometriosis. However, reports of the use of robotic-assisted surgery to treat this condition are limited but do demonstrate the feasibility of this technique (Jenkins 2004; Nezhat et al. 2006).

8.7. Oncology

Laparoscopy has been used in gynecologic oncology surgery for staging and treatment of early-stage endometrial cancer (Barakat 2005; Yu et al. 2005; Janda et al. 2006; Willis et al. 2006; Kalogiannidis et al. 2007; Nezhat et al. 2007). The radical gynecologic procedures also lend themselves to robotic-assisted surgical techniques. These procedures are usually performed through large debilitating wounds with significant morbidity. Hence this patient population would benefit most from this technology.

Marchal et al. (2005) published their series of gynecologic oncology consisting of 12 cases (seven cervical and five endometrial cancers). The mean lymph-node harvest was 11 (range 4–21). At a mean follow-up of 10 months (range 4–21) no recurrences were noted. Reynolds et al. (2005) conducted a smaller study of seven patients consisting of four endometrial, two ovarian, and one fallopian tube cancer. The median lymph node harvest was 15 (range 4–29).

Guru et al. (2007) have reported anterior exenteration in urologic surgery for bladder cancer. This is not directly comparable to anterior exenteration in gynecologic oncology as this procedure is performed for cervical or endometrial cancer recurrence following radiotherapy treatment. However, the seven cases presented do illustrate the feasibility of this surgery. In these cases the uterus was dissected and mobilized first, then the vascular pedicles were secured (superior vesicle, and the branches of the anterior internal iliac branch) followed by vaginal dissection. The bladder was mobilized and urethra dissected and the specimen removed through the introitus. The uterus was then removed; and the vagina reconstructed. Urinary diversion or reconstruction were performed extracorporeally through a midline incision. To anastomose the neobladder to the urethra, the neobladder was placed in the pelvis, the abdominal wound closed, and anastomosis performed with robotic assistance.

8.8. Pelvic Reconstructive Surgery

8.8.1. Sacrocolpopexy

It is estimated that almost one in nine women undergo hysterectomy in their life time (Marchionni et al. 1999). Of these 10% develop vaginal vault prolapse requiring surgical repair. Depending upon the individual's age, lifestyle, and comorbidities repair is performed through the transvaginal or transabdominal route. Of the two approaches, transabdominal sacrocolpopexy using synthetic meshes has yielded the most durable success rates and hence is the preferred choice of repair in relatively young patients who are in good general health. As long-term success rates of transvaginal repair are consistently inferior to transabdominal repair, transvaginal repair is reserved for patients who are not fit for major surgery (Benson et al. 1996). Laparoscopic sacrocolpopexy has failed to gain widespread acceptance because of the technical limitation of the technique and advanced expertise required to execute the procedure. However, robotic technology with its unique features is offering a suitable alternative. The largest series of sacrocolpopexy performed using robotic-assisted surgical techniques was recently published (Elliott et al. 2006). Thirty patients with posthysterectomy vault prolapse had robotic-assisted laparoscopic sacrocolpopexy at the Mayo Clinic. Ten patients also underwent a concurrent anti-incontinence procedure to treat urinary incontinence. Mean operating time was 3.1 hours (range 1.5–4.75 hours), with a mean hospital stay of one day. Twenty one had minimum follow-up of 12 months. One patient developed a recurrent grade-3 rectocele, another vault prolapse and two vaginal extrusions of the mesh. One patient developed recurrent vaginal vault prolapse at 24 months. Patients reported a high level of satisfaction. These investigators noted that the learning curve was an obvious limitation but technical difficulties associated with the procedure are reduced with the use of the robotic system.

Daneshgari et al. (2007) reported feasibility and short-term outcome of 15 cases of robotic abdominal sacrocolpopexy and sacrouteropexy for advanced pelvic organ prolapse, concluding that the technique is safe and its outcomes compare favorably with open or laparoscopic abdominal sacrocolpopexy. Patients were placed in low lithotomy position. They performed the procedure through five or six ports. The camera port (12 mm) was placed lateral to the umbilicus. Robotic ports were inserted at the midpoint of a line drawn between umbilicus and 2 cm above the anterior superior iliac spine on each side. A 12-mm port was placed lateral to the right robotic port and either one or two 5-mm ports were placed 2 cm above the anterior superior iliac spine. The robot was then docked. Intracorporeal dissection was performed and the mesh placed and sutured to the vaginal apex anteriorly and to the sacral promontory posteriorly. This was followed by closure of the peritoneum over the mesh. Of the 15 patients who agreed to have the procedure 12 had a successful procedure, whilst three required conversion to a different approach for various adverse intraoperative factors. Seven patients had concurrent placement of transobturator tape and one had a Burch colposuspension. The mean hospital stay was 2.4 days (range 1–7 days). All patients had good objective outcomes at 6 months follow-up, although functional outcomes were not assessed.

8.8.2. *Vesicovaginal Fistula Repair*

The first case of robotic-assisted vesicovaginal fistula repair was published by Melamud et al. in 2005. Sundaram et al. (2006) reported the technique of vesicovaginal repair and the results of such repairs in five patients. The proposed sequence of steps was similar to the open transabdominal repair of the fistula including excision of the fistula, closure of the bladder, and vagina and omental interposition. The mean operating time was 233 min (range 150–333 min) with an estimated blood loss of 70 ml and mean length of hospital stay of 5 days (range 4–7 days). All reported cases were completely dry at 6 months follow-up (100% cure rate).

8.9. Robotic Colposuspension

Surgery for stress urinary continence is still evolving. New concepts about pathophysiology of stress urinary incontinence have led to the introduction of mid-urethral tapes. These tapes have made surgical procedures simple and minimally invasive. Short- and medium-term outcomes are comparable to the accepted gold standard operation of open colposuspension (Ward et al. 2002).

Laparoscopy has been employed to offset the disadvantages of open colposuspension but the reported success rates have been variable (Moehrer et al. 2000). To perform a successful laparoscopic colposuspension the surgeon should ideally be ambidextrous with intracorporeal suturing–a skill not easy to master.

Robotic colposuspension offers an alternative to open and laparoscopic colposuspension. It is minimally invasive and the procedure emulates the open operation in all technical respects. Only two cases (Khan et al. 2007) of robotic colposuspension have been reported with one-year follow-up. One procedure was complicated by right ureteric kinking which required laparoscopic removal of the suspending sutures. This procedure though feasible is best performed as an adjunct in patients requiring other intrapelvic procedures who may suffer from genuine stress incontinence.

It is unlikely that robotic colposuspension will become the standard of care because of the high capital and disposable costs of the da Vinci^{TM} system. However, it is hoped that robotics will become cheaper over time making the procedure cost-efficient. In addition if the robotic system is already in place, cost of the disposables is largely offset by the well-known advantages of minimal invasive surgery like shorter hospital stay, reduced morbidity, and early return to the work. Thus, subject to the availability of the machine, robotic colposuspension may be regarded as an effective surgical treatment for patients requiring antistress incontinence surgery.

Patients are placed in a 45° Trendelenburg position and strapped to the operating table. The arms are kept by the patient's sides and gelfoam pads used throughout to protect pressure points. The legs are placed in stirrups to allow cystoscopy and vaginal access, with the hips being flexed. Criss-cross (X) strapping over gel pads is applied to the chest with care being taken to prevent any difficulty with respiratory excursions and prevent neuromuscular complications from undue compression at pressure points. Port positions are depicted in the diagram (Fig. 8.1).

Through an infraumbilical incision the extraperitoneal space is developed using balloon dissection. The robotic stereoscopic camera is introduced through a port placed through the same incision. Two 8-mm robotic ports are placed just lateral to the rectus abdominis along the line joining the anterior superior iliac spine to the umbilicus about 5 cm below the level of the umbilicus, on either side. A 10-mm assistant port is inserted about 5 cm above and medial to the right anterior superior iliac spine for suction and introduction of sutures. In obese patients it may be necessary to shift the ports downwards by a couple of cm to allow ease of pelvic access. In these cases measuring port sites in relation to the symphysis pubis as a fixed point rather than the umbilicus may be more useful. The da Vinci™ system is then attached to the patient and docked. Robotic instruments are used to clear the space of Retzius of fat and expose the paravaginal tissues, lateral margins of the bladder, and Cooper's ligaments. Three sutures of '0'Ethibond are placed between the paravaginal tissues at the bladder neck and the Cooper's ligament on each side using square to slip knot technique. The tension on the sutures is adjusted by the assistant lifting the ipsilateral lateral fornix with a Hegar dilator inserted vaginally. A drain is left in situ to avoid any retroperitoneal collection and removed the next morning.

As in open surgery it is important to check cystoscopically to make sure that the sutures have not transgressed the bladder. Ureteric compression from kinking or even accidental ligation is possible albeit rare as the ureters are not visible during the procedure. Careful delineation of the lateral margins of the bladder may reduce this risk. Placement of sutures on the ileo-pectineal Cooper's ligament can be technically challenging and we suggest holding the needle nearer the tip to ease this part of the procedure.

The average operating time was 145 min, docking time 6 min. The operating time was somewhat longer probably as this was a new procedure. Average blood loss was 15 ml. Postoperatively each patient required a total of 15 mg of morphine. Both patients were able to void postoperatively with minimal residual volumes. Total hospital stay was 2 days for one patient and 7 days for the other. The prolonged stay in the second patient was due to postoperative right ureteric obstruction caused by kinking of the right ureter by the most lateral suture. The suture had not gone through the ureter and was not visible in the bladder, which had been checked cystoscopically. It had caused ureteric kinking most likely due to increased pull and tension on it while it was being tied. This was recognized and managed by subsequent laparoscopic suture division through the existing port sites. At follow-up of 6 and 12 months both patients were continent.

8.10. Robotic vs. Laparoscopic Gynecology

Robotics in gynecology has several advantages over conventional laparoscopy (Table 8.3). Tissue handling and suturing have been noted to be much easier because of the unique instrument design. Greater degrees-of-freedom of movement and three-dimensional viewing contribute to a less-steep learning curve compared to conventional laparoscopy.

The da Vinci^{TM} robot is still in the second generation of its production, and as it was designed specifically for cardiac surgery the engineers did not consider the requirements of abdominal surgery. The instrumentation is limited and the robotic arms bulky and not attached to the operating room table. Large excursions of the arms can lead to collision. The strong robotic arms lack tensile feedback. Thus, use of the telerobot in the standard operating rooms is cumbersome and frustrating. An additional drawback in relation to gynecologic surgery is the lack of vaginal access. Equipment cost is an issue with sums totalling 1.4 million dollars, annual maintenance and instrument usage also adding to this. In addition, the extra theatre time and training of personnel needs to be assessed.

8.11. Conclusions

The landscape of robotic surgery has changed dramatically and modified our view of the role of the robot in surgical practice over the last 5 years. The current technology has amalgamated the enhancements in computer-aided 3-D imaging,

TABLE 8.3 Comparison of laparoscopic and robotic-assisted minimally invasive surgery

	Conventional laparoscopy	Robotic-assisted surgery
Visualization	2D and unsteady	3D and steady
Laparoscope control	Manual	Mechanical
Instruments	Rigid	Articulated, Endowrist instruments
Degrees-of-movement	Three degrees-of-movement	Seven degrees-of-movement
Hand movement	Counter-intuitive	Intuitive
Instrument movement	Direct	Downscaled
Tactile feedback (haptics)	Reduced	Reduced
Tremor	Yes	No
Set up time	Relatively quick	Longer
Learning curve	Steep for complex procedures	Shorter for complex surgery
Training staff	Usually staff already trained	Extra training required
Complex surgery	Access, visualization, and degrees-of-movement hamper surgery	May allow for more complex surgery
Cost	Absorbed within departments	May be prohibitively expensive
Remote surgery	No	Yes

engineering feats such as the endoscopic manipulator and laparoscopic technology. This has transformed the status of robotic surgery from that of an experimental procedure to possible routine practice in many surgical disciplines including gynecology. As a majority of gynecologists have experience of conventional laparoscopy the potential to transfer those skills to robotics is clearly present and the benefit to patients potentially enormous.

Obvious shortcomings of the current robotic systems include high cost, bulkiness of the apparatus, and lack of tactile feedback but it is expected that future developments will focus on refining haptic feedback, system miniaturization, improved augmented reality and telesurgical capabilities. Any gynecologic procedure suitable for laparoscopic surgery should in theory be amenable to robotic-assisted surgery if the facilities and expertise are available. However, only through prospective trials comparing robotics to standard laparoscopic surgery can this new technology be fully evaluated.

References

Advincula AP, Song A, Burke W, Reynolds RK (2004) Preliminary experience with robot-assisted laparoscopic myomectomy. J Am Assoc Gynecol Laparosc 11 (4):511–518

Advincula AP, Reynolds RK (2005) The use of robot-assisted laparoscopic hysterectomy in the patient with a scarred or obliterated anterior culdesac. J Soc Laparoendosc Surg 9:287–291

Advincula AP (2006) Surgical techniques: robot-assisted laparoscopic hysterectomy with the da Vinci surgical system. Int J Med Robotics Comput Assist Surg 2:305–311

Advincula AP, Song A (2007) The role of robotic surgery in gynecology 2007. Curr Opin Obstet Gynecol 19:331–336

Barakat RR (2005) Laparoscopic assisted staging for endometrial cancer. Int J Gynecol Cancer 15 (2):407

Benson JT, Lucente V, McLellan E (1996) Vaginal versus abdominal reconstructive surgery for the treatment of pelvic support defects: a prospective randomised study with long-term evaluation. Am J Obstet Gynecol 175:418

Beste TM, Nelson KH, Daucher JA (2005) Total laparoscopic hysterectomy utilizing a robotic surgical system. J Soc Laparoendosc Surg 9:13–15

Bisharah M, Tulandi T (2003) Laparoscopic preservation of ovarian function: an underused procedure. Am J Obstet Gynecol 188:367–370

Cadiere GB, Himpens J, Germay O, Izizaw R, Degueldre M, Vandromme J, Capelluto E, Bruyns J (2001) Feasibility of robotic laparoscopic surgery: 146 cases. World J Surg 25:1467–1477

Daneshgari F, Kefer CJ, Moore C, Kaouk J (2007) Robotic abdominal sacro-colpopexy/sacrouteropexy repair of advanced female pelvic organ prolapse (POP): utilizing POP-quantification based staging and outcomes. BJU Int 100:875–879

Degueldre M, Vandromme J, Huong PT, Cadiere GB (2000) Robotically assisted laparoscopic microsurgical tubal reanastamosis: a feasibility study. Fertil Steril 74:1020–1023

Diaz-Arrastia C, Jurnalov C, Gomez G, Townsend C Jr. (2002) Laparoscopic hysterectomy using a computer-enhanced surgical robot. Surg Endosc 16:1271–1273

Doridot V, Dubuisson JB, Chapron C, Fauconnier A, Babaki-Fard K et al. (2001) Recurrence of leiomyomata after laparoscopic myomectomy. J Am Assoc Gynecol Laparosc 8: 495–500

Elliott DS, Krambeck AE, Chow GK (2006) Long term results of robot-assisted laparoscopic sacrocolpopexy for the treatment of high grade vaginal vault prolapse. J Urol 176:655–659

Falcone T, Goldberg J, Garcia-Ruiz A, Margossian H, Stevens L (1999) Full robotic assistance for laparoscopic tubal anastamosis: a case report. J Laroendosc Adv Surg Tech A 9:107–113

Fiorentino RP, Zepeda M, Goldstein BH et al. (2006) Pilot study assessing robot laparoscopic hysterectomy and patient outcomes. J Minim Invasive Gynecol 13:60–63

Guru KA, Nogueira M, Piacente P, Nyquist J, Mohler JL, Kim HL (2007) Robot-assisted anterior exenteration: technique and initial series. J Endourol 21 (6):633–639

Janda M, Gebski V, Forder P, Jackson D, Williams G, Obermair A LACE Trial Committee (2006) Total laparoscopic versus open surgery for stage 1 endometrial cancer: the LACE randomized controlled trial. Contemp Clin Trials 27 (4):353–363

Jenkins TR (2004) Laparoscopic supracervical hysterectomy. Am J Obstet Gynecol 191 (6):1875–1884

Kalogiannidis I, Lambrechts S, Amant F, Neven P, Van Gorp T, Vergote I (2007) Laparoscopy-assisted vaginal hysterectomy compared with abdominal hysterectomy in clinical stage I endometrial cancer: safety, recurrence, and long-term outcome. Am J Obstet Gynecol 196 (3):248.e1–8

Kenney A, Papadopoulos AJ (2001) Uterine Fibroids. Curr Obstet Gynaecol 11 (5):285–295

Khan MS, Challacombe BJ, Rose K, Dasgupta P (2007) Robotic colposuspension: two case reports. J Endourol 21 (9): 1077–1079

Kho RM, Hilger WS, Hentz JG, Magtibay PM, Magrina JF (2007) Robotic hysterectomy: technique and initial outcomes. Am J Obstet Gynecol 197: 113e1–113e4

Mais V, Ajossa S, Guerriero S, Mascia M, Solla E, Melis GB (1996) Laparoscopic versus abdominal myomectomy: prospective randomised trial to evaluate benefits in early outcome. Am J Obstet Gynecol 174:654–658

Marchionni M, Bracco GL, Checcucci V, Carabaneanu A, Coccia EM, Mecacci F et al. (1999) True incidence of vaginal vault prolapse. Thirteen years of experience. J Reprod Med 44:679

Marchal F, Rauch P, Vandromme J, Laurent I, Lobontiu A, Ahcel B, Verhaeghe JL, Meistelman C, Degueldre M, Villemot JP, Guillemin F (2005) Telerobotic-assisted laparoscopic hysterectomy for benign and oncologic pathologies: initial clinical experience with 30 patients. Surg Endosc 19:826–831

Melamud O, Elehel L, Turbow et al. (2005) Laparoscopic vesicovaginal fistula repair with robotic reconstruction. Urology 65: 163–166

Moehrer B et al. (2000) Laparoscopic colpo-suspension for urinary incontinence in women. The Cochrane Database of Systemic Reviews Issue 3. Art No:CD00239

Molpus KL, Wedegren JS, Carlson MA (2003) Robotically assisted endoscopic ovarian transposition. J Soc Laparoendosc Surg 7: 59–62

Nezhat C, Siegler A, Nezhat F, Nezhat C, Siedman D, Luciano A (2000) Operative Gynecologic Laparoscopy; Principles and Techniques, 2nd Ed. McGraw Hill, New York

Nezhat C, Saberi NS, Shahmohamady B, Nezhat F (2006) Robotic-assisted Laparoscopy: in gynecological surgery. J Soc Laparoendosc Surg 10:317–320

Nezhat F, Prasad Hayes M, Peiretti M, Rahaman J (2007) Laparoscopic radical parametrectomy and partial vaginectomy for recurrent endometrial cancer. Gynecol Oncol 104 (2):494–496

Olive DL, Parker WH, Cooper JM, Levine RL (2000) The American association of gynaecologic laparoscopists classification system for laparoscopic hysterectomy. Classification committee of the American association of gynaecologic laparoscopists. J Am Assoc Gynecol Laparosc 7:9–15

Raju KS, Auld BJ (1994) A randomised prospective study of laparoscopic vaginal hysterectomy versus abdominal hysterectomy each with bilateral salpingo-oophorectomy. Br J Obstet Gynaecol 101 (12):1068–1071

Reynolds RK, Burke WM, Advincula AP (2005) Preliminary experience with robot-assisted laparoscopic staging of gynaecologic malignancies. J Soc Laparoendosc Surg 9(2):149–158

Reynolds RK, Advincula AP (2006) Robot-assisted laparoscopic hysterectomy: technique and initial experience. Am J Surg 191:555–560

Senapati S, Advincula AP (2007) Surgical techniques: robot-assisted laparoscopic myomectomy with the da Vinci surgical system. J Robot Surg 1:69–74

Seracchioli R, Rossi S, Govoni F, Rossi E, Venturoli S, Bulletti C, Flamigni C (2000) Fertility and obstetric outcome after laparoscopic myomectomy of large myomata: a randomised comparison with abdominal myomectomy. Hum Reprod 15:2663–2668

Sundaram BM, Kalidasan G, Hemal AK (2006) Robotic repair of vesicovaginal fistula: a case series of 5 patients. Urology 65 (5):970–973

Styolopoulos N, Rattner D (2003) Robotics and ergonomics. Surg Clin North Am 83:1321–1337

Yu CK, Cutner A, Mould T, Olaitian A (2005) Total laparoscopic hysterectomy as a primary surgical treatment for endometrial cancer in morbidly obese women. Br J Obstet Gynecol 112 (1):115–117

Ward KL et al. on behalf of the UK TVT Trial Group (2002) Prospective multi-centre randomized controlled trial of tension-free vaginal tape and colpo-suspension as primary treatment for stress urinary incontinence. Br Med J 325:67–70

Willis SF, Barton D, Ind TE (2006) Laparoscopic hysterectomy with or without pelvic lymphadenectomy or sampling in a high-risk series of patients with endometrial cancer. Int Semin Surg Oncol 13 (3):28

Chapter 9
Anesthesia
and Robotic-Assisted Surgery

Lisa Blake, Marcin Sicinski, and Sanjay Gulati

Abstract: Robotic surgery presents unique anesthetic challenges. The bulkiness of the equipment combined with steep Trendelenburg position and pneumoperitoneum demands close attention to detail to avoid complications. Careful patient positioning, attention to intubation and ventilation and awareness of a rise in intracranial pressure are crucial to success. Enhanced patient recovery programs can shorten the post-operative stay.

Keywords: Anesthesia, Trendelenburg, positive end expiratory pressure, pneumoperitoneum, enhanced recovery

9.1. Introduction

Urology remains at the forefront of minimally invasive surgery. In no other specialty has the arrival of robotic technology in particular, been greeted with such enthusiasm. The da Vinci^TM surgical system (Intuitive Surgical, Sunnyvale, California) is the principal surgical robot in current use. The technical features of this robot are described elsewhere in this book. Robotic-assisted laparoscopic radical prostatectomy (RALP) using the da Vinci^TM system is the most commonly performed robotic procedure worldwide, and during

P. Dasgupta (ed.), *Robotic Urological Surgery in Clinical Practice*, 181
DOI: 10.1007/978-1-84800-243-2_9,
© Springer-Verlag London Limited 2008

2007 accounted for about 60% of radical prostatectomies in the USA.

The increasing use of this technology raises particular issues for anesthesia requirements during robotic-assisted surgery. Apart from the physiologic changes associated with prolonged pneumoperitoneum and certain patient positions, the bulky nature of this technology restricts access to the patient and prevents adjustments to patient position once the robot has been docked. This chapter reviews these challenges from an anesthetic perspective.

9.2. Robotic-Assisted Laparoscopic Urology

Urologists now routinely use a laparoscopic approach for the following procedures:

- Simple and radical nephrectomy.
- Nephroureterectomy.
- Pyeloplasty.
- Radical prostatectomy.
- Pelvic lymph-node dissection.

In specialized units radical cystectomy and urinary diversion are also undertaken laparoscopically. The surgical approach may be extra- or transperitoneal for many of these procedures. An extraperitoneal approach may limit complications related to pneumoperitoneum such as shoulder-tip pain and decreased venous return. However, the majority of robotic-assisted laparoscopic procedures are performed by a transperitoneal approach, so for the purposes of discussion we will presume this approach for the following chapter.

9.3. Physiology of Laparoscopic Surgery

Many of the procedures listed above involve anesthesia times of 3 hours or more. Therefore, the consequences of prolonged pneumoperitoneum and certain patient positions need to be considered and planned for (Gerges et al. 2006). As in other types of laparoscopic surgery, carbon dioxide (CO_2) is used for insufflation. For urologic procedures, the intraabdominal pressure is maintained at 12–15 mmHg. The potential physiologic changes associated with CO_2 pneumoperitoneum include:

- Decreased functional residual capacity.
- Decreased compliance.
- Ventilation/perfusion mismatch.
- Increased shunting due to atelectasis.
- Hypercapnia due to CO_2 absorption.
- Increased pulmonary vascular resistance.
- Elevated arterial pressures.
- Decreased cardiac output.

Though some of the changes listed above may have a negligible effect on the induction and maintenance of safe anesthesia in a healthy patient, additional factors may be present which may exacerbate such changes. For laparoscopic radical prostatectomy and laparoscopic radical cystectomy, a steep Trendelenburg position is usually required (see Fig. 9.1). This, combined with the pneumoperitoneum, can lead to a

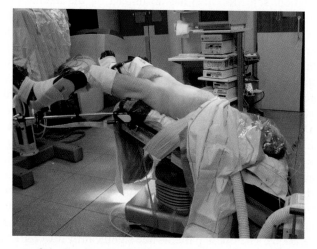

FIGURE 9.1. A steep Trendelenburg position is usually required for RALP.

fall in cardiac output of 10–30% (Joris 2005). This is secondary to decreased venous return from caval compression and dependent venous pooling. Surgeons occasionally ask for the pneumoperitoneum to be raised to decrease troublesome venous oozing. The maximum setting allowed on most laparoscopic insufflators is 20 mmHg. The anesthetic team should be informed of such changes in pneumoperitoneum and the intraabdominal pressure should be returned to the standard setting as soon as feasible to avoid decreased venous return.

Prolonged pneumoperitoneum may restrict respiratory excursion due to cephalad displacement of the diaphragm. This may lead to decreased arterial oxygenation and atelectasis. A study from Scandinavia examined whether the addition of positive end expiratory pressure (PEEP) could improve arterial oxygenation during robotic-assisted laparoscopic radical prostatectomy, compared to standard mechanical ventilation (Meininger et al. 2005). In a group of 20 men undergoing RALP, ten were randomized to receive standard mechanical ventilation, while ten received 5-cm H_2O in addition. The addition of PEEP resulted in increased arterial oxygenation during prolonged pneumoperitoneum.

Patient selection also has an impact on the likelihood of physiologic sequelae during laparoscopic procedures. By definition, men being considered for radical prostatectomy are less than 70 years of age with reasonable performance status. The same cannot be said of those undergoing radical cystectomy who are often older with smoking-related risk factors. Obesity, defined as those with body mass index (BMI) >30 kg/m^2, is also becoming an issue for many patient populations in the Western World, including those undergoing robotic surgery. Airway management and patient positioning are more challenging in this group, who have a higher surgical and anesthetic complication rate compared to those with BMI <30 kg/m^2 (Passannante and Rock 2005). Meininger et al. studied a group of 15 obese men undergoing RALP and compared their anesthetic management to a similar group of 15 nonobese men (Meininger et al. 2006). The obese patients had significantly lower arterial oxygenation during pneumoperitoneum though no long-term consequences were noted.

Specific complications related to the intraperitoneal insufflation of carbon dioxide include (Pathan and Gulati 2007):

- Subcutaneous emphysema.
- Pneumothorax.
- Endobronchial intubation.
- Gas embolism.

Of these, subcutaneous emphysema is a not uncommon and not serious consequence of CO_2 diffusing into the soft tissues outside the abdominal cavity. Pneumothorax may be caused by surgical perforation of the diaphragm during laparoscopic renal surgery. However, this is rare in robotic-assisted surgery as the large majority of procedures involve pelvic organs. Spontaneous rupture of bullae in patients with pre-existing obstructive pulmonary disease is a rare cause of pneumothorax in laparoscopic urology. Endobronchial intubation may occur as a result of cephalad movement of the diaphragm once pneumoperitoneum is established, especially in those patients with a steep Trendelenburg position. We have noted an unusual variation of this situation with obstruction of the endotracheal (ET) tube due to pneumoperitoneum by abutting against the trachea itself.

Gas embolism is a very rare but potentially catastrophic complication of CO_2 insufflation. Simple diffusion of CO_2 into the vascular system is not sufficient to cause the sudden cardiorespiratory deterioration seen with gas embolism. Rather, a large amount of gas must be infused under high pressure directly into a large vessel, a quite unlikely event with modern laparoscopic techniques.

9.4. Specific Issues with Robotic-Assisted Surgery

The arrival of the da Vinci™ surgical system has introduced new challenges to the anesthetic team in the urology theatre. The technology is discussed in detail elsewhere in this book.

Briefly, the da Vinci™ system is composed of three components:

1. *Surgeon's console*: The surgeon controls the robot from a console placed away from the operating table. The surgeon's thumb and forefinger control the movements of the robotic arms.
2. *Patient-side cart*: the robotic "arms" are mounted on this 600 kg cart, one of which holds the high-resolution 3D endoscope. The arms are bolted or "docked" to the patient, greatly restricting patient repositioning.
3. *Image-processing/insufflation stack*: the stack contains the camera-control units for the 3-D imaging system, image-recording devices, a laparoscopic insufflator, and a monitor allowing 2D vision for the assistants.

In addition to the specific physiologic issues of laparoscopic surgery discussed above, the presence of a somewhat bulky and immovable object, bolted to the unconscious patient, poses some new challenges (see Fig. 9.2).

Firstly, the robotic cart presents a formidable obstacle between the anesthetic team and the patient. This is less so for pelvic surgery when the cart is positioned between the patient's legs, but for renal surgery it may be parked close to the head end of the table. The anesthetic machine and ancillary equipment may have to be relocated. The cart is "docked" to the patient using three or four specialized ports preventing repositioning of the patient. In an emergency situation it may take a little time to undock the robot and remove it from the patient-side. This engagement between the patient and robotic cart also may lead to potential injury caused by inadvertent patient movement.

Secondly, the cart itself should not be in contact with the patient save for its docked position to the robotic ports. However, it is in close proximity to the patient's legs during pelvic surgery and care must be taken to ensure it is not in contact at these points. There is no haptic feedback through the robotic arms and inadvertent pressure injury could occur at these points.

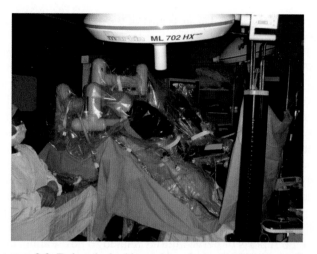

FIGURE 9.2. Robot docked in position during RALP. The patient's head is towards the right of the picture, concealed under drapes. Note the steep Trendelenburg position.

Thirdly, the principal surgeon is located away from the patient-side—a quite new concept in laparoscopic surgery. Clear lines of communication must exist between the console and patient-side surgeons to compensate for this layout. An intercom system is integrated into the da Vinci™ system which helps in this regard.

Despite these challenges, the system appears to function in a safe and efficacious manner. Costello et al. evaluated their early experience with the da Vinci™ from an anesthetic perspective (Costello and Webb 2006). Their series of 40 patients underwent RALP using the da Vinci™ system. Epidural anesthesia was used in 26 of these patients, who were noted to have less opiate analgesia requirements on the postoperative period. No specific complications related to the laparoscopic or robotic technique were noted. The overall hospital stay for the group was 4.2 days, compared with 8.2 days for open radical prostatectomy patients in their region. We no longer employ epidural analgesia as part of the anesthetic technique at our institution.

The world's largest robotic surgery center has also reported its experience of RALP from an anesthetic perspective. Danic et al. reviewed their first 1500 cases and reported no deaths and very few complications (Danic et al. 2007). The most common surgical complication was ileus which occurred in 1.7% of patients and usually settled with conservative management. The reoperation rate for their series was 0.6%. Blood transfusion was required in 1% of patients. Interestingly, the most commonly reported anesthetic-related complication was corneal abrasion which occurred in 3% of patients despite the use of eye tape. Three patients (0.2%) developed pulmonary emboli requiring anticoagulation. Of note, there were no reports of nerve injuries related to positioning, or of cardiorespiratory complications related to the pneumoperitoneum.

However, some case reports are emerging of complications attributed to robotic-assisted laparoscopic surgery. Phong et al. report two specific problems they encountered during da Vinci™-assisted surgery (Phong and Koh 2007). The first case required emergency reintubation following robotic-assisted laparoscopic radical prostatectomy due to laryngeal edema. This was attributed to decreased venous return and prolonged Trendelenburg positioning. The second case was mild brachial plexus neuropraxia which resolved spontaneously. This was clearly related to the shoulder brace used to maintain the patient on the table while in the extreme Trendelenburg position.

9.5. Anesthetic Technique

Safe provision of anesthesia for robotic urology requires a well-planned multidisciplinary approach.

Preoperative assessment will necessarily concentrate on the cardiovascular and respiratory systems and any renal dysfunction should also be noted. Outpatient preassessment screening allows time for preoperative investigations and planning. Patients presenting for urologic procedures often suffer significant and multiple comorbidities and may require further investigations before formulating an appropriate anesthetic plan. Evaluation of functional status by cardiopulmonary exercise testing can be particularly useful in informing decisions on borderline patients. A number of special considerations apply when assessing an obese patient (BMI $>30 \, kg/m^2$), particularly in terms of higher risk of cardiovascular and respiratory comorbidities. The combination of steep Trendelenburg position and pneumoperitoneum may lead to potential problems in maintaining adequate ventilation and avoiding barotrauma.

The choice of anesthetic technique used for urologic robotic surgery must take in to account several important factors associated with this type of surgery.

9.5.1. Airway and Ventilation

Patient position, length of surgery, and pneumoperitoneum makes endotracheal intubation mandatory. Pulmonary compliance is reduced and higher ventilation pressures are required to maintain adequate tidal volume. In addition, absorption of carbon dioxide used to produce the pneumoperitoneum may lead to hypercapnia. Permissive hypercapnia is not recommended as there will be an additive effect with the Trendelenburg position on intracranial pressure. Pressure control ventilation and manipulation of I:E time ratios should allow for adequate ventilation without excessive risk of barotrauma, except in those with severe pre-existing respiratory disease.

9.5.2. Cardiovascular Stability and Fluid Management

Cardiac output is generally reduced, and the effect on arterial pressure can be variable. In addition, intravenous fluids should be restricted to minimize facial and possibly cerebral edema. Reduction of urine output is also beneficial to allow a better surgical field prior to completion of the urethrovesical anastomosis. Vigorous fluid infusion is then commenced, to optimize cardiac output, following completion of the anastomosis.

9.5.3. Intracranial Pressure

There are some concerns regarding raised intracranial pressure during surgery due to the position of the patient and reduction in venous return secondary to raised intra-abdominal pressure. In addition, if cerebral autoregulation is impaired from hypercapnia and operative times are prolonged, then this may become clinically relevant. In our early experience, when operative times were longer, we did see instances of confusion in the early postoperative period, and a short period of elective postoperative ventilation can be considered in difficult cases.

On one occasion, we have seen some evidence of raised intracranial pressure on Entropy monitoring. The use of Entropy as an intracranial pressure monitor is not established. The patient recovered with no sequelae in this instance following a short period of elective ventilation (Hornero et al. 2006).

9.5.4. Analgesia

Because of the minimally invasive approach of robotic surgery, the use of epidurals for pain management is not generally recommended. We have good experience at this institution with the use of caudal epidurals for postoperative analgesia for RALP. Intrathecal diamorphine is a useful technique for pyeloplasty and nephrectomy.

Epidurals are useful in the management of patients undergoing cystectomy and ileal conduit formation. The sympathetic blockade also reduces the incidence of postoperative ileus.

9.5.5. Monitoring

Routine basic monitoring, including temperature is adequate for most patients undergoing the majority of robotic-assisted procedures. One 14–16G cannula should provide adequate i.v. access.

Invasive monitoring should be reserved for patients with significant comorbidities and should certainly be considered in patients undergoing cystectomy. We do not routinely employ central venous monitoring for robotic-assisted cystectomies, although we do then use oesophageal Doppler cardiac output measurement. It may also be beneficial to initially use invasive monitoring techniques in institutions introducing robotic programs, where prolonged operative times are expected.

9.6. Enhanced Recovery after Surgery

When patients are assessed for surgery, there is usually an intervening period of some weeks prior to surgery. This may allow some lifestyle interventions, where motivated patients may undertake appropriate physical activity, modify diet, decrease alcohol intake, and attempt smoking cessation, if relevant.

We have also introduced some of the principles of *enhanced recovery after surgery*, which are now established in both open and laparoscopic colorectal surgery. Psychologic preparation for early discharge starts at the preoperative visit (Fearon et al. 2005; Kehlet and Wilmore 2002).

Preoperative fasting is minimized, and bowel preparation and postoperative nasogastric drainage are not employed. Regional anesthesia is used as appropriate, high inspired oxygen concentrations are used intraoperatively and early postoperative feeding and mobilization are encouraged.

9.7. Conclusions

The advent of robotic-assisted laparoscopic surgery has provided some interesting challenges for the anesthetist. These relate primarily to the patient positioning, prolonged pneumoperitoneum, and the actual robotic equipment itself.

A coordinated team approach to this surgery has allowed this form of surgery to be successfully introduced at our institution with excellent patient acceptance and satisfaction. Modifying the perioperative management to account for these challenges allows patients to be discharged early following surgery and aids early recovery.

References

Costello TG, Webb P (2006) Anesthesia for robot-assisted anatomic prostatectomy. Experience at a single Institution. Anaesth Intensive Care 34(6):787–792

Danic MJ, Chow M, Alexander G, Bhandari A, Menon M, Brown M (2007) Anesthesia concerns for robotic-assisted laparoscopic prostatectomy: a review of 1,500 cases. J Robotic Surg 1(2): 119–123

Fearon KC, Ljungqvist O, Von Meyenfeldt M, Revhaug A, Dejong CH, Lassen K, Nygren J, Hausel J, Soop M, Andersen J, Kehlet H (2005) Enhanced recovery after surgery: a consensus review of clinical care for patients undergoing colonic resection. Clin Nutr 24(3):466–477. Epub 2005 Apr 21

Hornero R, Aboy M, Abasolo D, McNames J, Wakeland W, Goldstein B (2006) Complex analysis of intracranial hypertension using approximate entropy. Crit Care Med 34(1)

Gerges FJ, Kanazi GE, Jabbour-Khoury SI (2006) Anesthesia for laparoscopy: a review. J Clin Anesth 18(1):67–78

Joris J (2005) Anesthesia for laparoscopic surgery. In: Miller R (ed) Anesthesia, 6th edn, chap. 57. Elsevier, Philadelphia

Kehlet H, Wilmore DW (2002) Multimodal strategies to improve surgical outcome. Am J Surg 183(6):630–641

Meininger D, Byhahn C, Mierdl S, Westphal K, Zwissler B (2005) Positive end-expiratory pressure improves arterial oxygenation during prolonged pneumoperitoneum. Acta Anaesthesiol Scand 49(6):778–783

Meininger D, Zwissler B, Byhahn C, Probst M, Westphal K, Bremerich DH (2006) Impact of overweight and pneumoperitoneum on hemodynamics and oxygenation during prolonged laparoscopic surgery. World J Surg 30(4):520–526

Passannante AN, Rock P (2005) Anesthetic management of patients with obesity and sleep apnea. Anesthesiol Clin North America 23(3):479–491, vii

Pathan H, Gulati S (2007) A case of airway occlusion in robotic surgery. J Robotic Surg 1(2):169–170

Phong SV, Koh LK (2007) Anesthesia for robotic-assisted radical prostatectomy: considerations for laparoscopy in the Trendelenburg position. Anaesth Intensive Care 35(2):281–285

Chapter 10
Health Economics of Robotic Surgery

Qing Wang, David Armstrong, and Alistair McGuire

Abstract: This chapter is focused on the economic evaluation of robotic surgery. Economic evaluation in healthcare programmes is defined as the "comparative analysis of alternative courses of action in terms of both their costs and consequences" (Drummond et al. 1997), and it aims to "ensure that benefits gained outweigh benefits forgone" [William (1986) in Drummond et al. (1997)].

In recent years, economic evaluation of healthcare programmes has increased in popularity to the point where it has become an indispensible part of any healthcare-related studies. The most widespread application of this subject is in the pharmaceutical industry, i.e., pharmaeconomics. The reasons of its increased application may be due to the recognition of the conflict between the limited health resources and unlimited health service demand. Economic evaluation can help in health service decision making, in health policy making, and in regulation of the healthcare market, where asymmetric information is abundant and free market access is prohibited.

This chapter considers the importance of the economic evaluation of robotic surgery and reviews the current state-of-art in this area. When new technologies involve substantial investment, economic evaluation can be used to establish a rational resource allocation system within a limited budget. Finally, this chapter concludes by making suggestions for

P. Dasgupta (ed.), *Robotic Urological Surgery in Clinical Practice*,   195
DOI: 10.1007/978-1-84800-243-2_10,
© Springer-Verlag London Limited 2008

future developments in the economic evaluation of robotic surgery.

Keywords: Economics, Evaluation, Decision modeling

10.1. The Importance of Economic Evaluation of Robotic Surgery

Increasing costs and demand for healthcare interventions, combined with limited resources and an imperfect market mechanism for resource allocation, has led to an increased interest in the economic evaluation of healthcare programmes. Economic evaluation in healthcare is the "comparative analysis of alternative courses of action in terms of both their costs and consequences" (Drummond et al. 1997).

As an alternative tool to the market mechanism (where the price of any good or service is the equilibrium point at which supply and demand are balanced), health economic evaluation has been developed to facilitate optimal resource allocation in those areas, such as healthcare, in which supply and demand do not operate in an unimpeded way (McGuire 2006).

Health economic evaluation studies are thriving worldwide, and gradually have become a mandatory component of any healthcare-related studies. In Sweden, for example, the Pharmaceutical Benefits Board, established in 2002, has required pharmaceutical manufacturers to submit health economic evaluations as part of their applications for reimbursement. In Australia, Canada, and the US, a similar requirement has been placed on pharmaceutical companies (Commonwealth of Australia 1995; FDA 1997; Anis and Gagnon 2000). The UK National Institute for Clinical Excellence (NICE) has adopted guidelines for the formal economic modeling in technology appraisals (NICE 2004).

However, despite these efforts and requirements, economic evaluation in surgery is still rare, and it is even less common in robotic surgery (Krahn 1999; Tooher and Pham

2004). Whilst the basic components of economic evaluation might be the same for every discipline, robotic surgery has features which require special consideration.

Robotic surgery is one of the most advanced techniques in minimal invasive surgery (MIS), and it is deemed by some surgeons as the future of surgery. Its clinical importance has been elaborated by professionals in previous chapters; and in this chapter, using the management of prostate surgery as an example, the importance, the challenges, and the development of economic evaluation of robotic surgery is demonstrated.

New medical technology such as robotic surgery involves substantial investment, and thus has significant implications on allocation of financial resources to healthcare. Currently, robotic surgery is more expensive to obtain, to maintain, and to perform, compared to the conventional alternatives. The additional cost arises from the development of the newer functions and more advanced facilities, such as 3D visualization and six degrees-of-freedom of robotic arms.

The next step in an economic evaluation would be to take the benefits of the new technology, convert these into a common currency, and compare these with the known costs of the technology. This step is the most difficult as the evidence for proclaimed "advantages" brought by these techniques is insufficient or biased. Further, the opportunity cost of new technologies, that is the alternative care that could be provided in its place with the resources it commands, has seldom been explored.

It has been reported that the cost of purchasing a da Vinci[TM] Robot system was $1.2 million, and the annual maintenance fee was $100,000 (Lotan et al. 2004). Therefore, it is important to conduct economic evaluation to establish a rational resource allocation system given the limited financial resources available for healthcare. Table 10.1. compares the current costs of open, laparoscopic, and robotic prostatectomy surgery in the United States at 2004 prices.

Establishment of cost relies on appropriate definition of episode length and in particular definition of the appropriate

TABLE 10.1. Hospital costs of open, laparoscopic, and robotic prostatectomy

Cost items	Open ($)	Laparoscopic ($)	Robotic (maintenance cost only) ($)	Robotic (purchase and maintenance costs) ($)
Operating room	2,428	2,867	2,204	2,204
Equipment	75	533	1,705	1,705
Surgeon fee	1,594	1,688	1,688	1,688
Hospital stay	988	514	474	474
Medications	150	78	72	72
Robot purchase and maintenance	NA	NA	286	857
Total	5,554	6,041	6,709	7,280

Source: Reproduced by the author from Lotan et al. (2004)

postoperative follow-up period. Information of readmission rates may be particularly difficult to observe in new technologies. The appropriate time frame for the analysis may also be dictated by the costs if the investment costs are associated with particular equipment. The capital costs must be apportioned over the appropriate lifetime of the equipment. Thus, the investment costs may determine the time frame of the analysis. In particular some form of estimate must be made of the timeframe over which capital costs will depreciate.

All economic evaluation requires evidence on clinical effectiveness. With surgery the establishment of such benefit is problematic. Generally, randomized clinical trials are difficult to perform as choice of comparator populations may be problematic, with most trials in surgery relying on head-to-head comparison of two interventions. Length of follow-up is a common issue, as is the fact that surgery may involve complex multifactorial intervention. Furthermore, the learning curve associated with new techniques means that the timing and location of such trials is important.

Not surprisingly the main benefits of robotic surgery, in terms of its clinical effectiveness, have yet to be established. Although some recent evidence has shown the promising future of robotic surgery, the evidence of its long-term efficacy is still incomplete (Tewari et al. 2006; Ficarra et al. 2007; Caceres et al. 2007). A systematic review (Tooher and Pham 2004) compared the efficacy and safety aspects of robotic surgery with those of open and conventional laparoscopic surgery, the results of which are shown in Table 10.2.

Because of the lack of evidence of the clinical advantage of robotic surgery, in combination with the substantial investment relating to purchasing, maintenance, and training, the NHS and major public hospitals are cautious in adopting this technology. In contrast with the US private healthcare market, the UK only has six public hospital centers that can supply the da Vinci[TM] robotic surgery service to patients. Since the NHS standard tariff only covers the cost of open surgery, which is roughly one third of the cost of robotic surgery, Primary Care Trusts are reluctant to assign extra funding for

TABLE 10.2. Key efficacy and safety results of robotic versus conventional surgery (conventional surgery: open or laparoscopic surgery)

Conventional procedures	Operative time	LOS	Conversions	Blood loss	Complications	Study
Open prostatectomy	Robotic longer (sig)	Robotic shorter (sig)	NR	Robotic less (Sig)	Robotic less (Not Sig)	Menon et al. 2002
Laparoscopic pyeloplasty	Robotic shorter (not sig)	Similar	NR	Similar	No complications	Gettman et al. 2002
Open coronary artery bypass grafting	NR	Robotic shorter (sig)	NR	NR	NR	Bucerius et al. 2002
Laparoscopic cholecystectomy	Robotic longer (not sig)	Robotic shorter (sig)	1	NR	Robotic less (not sig)	Giulianotti et al. 2003
Laparoscopic fundoplication	Robotic shorter (not sig)	Robotic shorter (sig)	0	NR	Robotic less (sig)	Giulianotti et al. 2003

Laparoscopic Fundoplication	Robotic longer (sig)	Similar	NR	NR	Similar	Melvin et al. 2002
Laparoscopic gastric banding	Robotic longer (not sig)	Similar	0	NR	No complications	Muhlmann et al. 2003
Open gastrectomy	Robotic longer (sig)	Similar	1	NR	Similar	Giulianotti et al. 2003
Laparoscopic/open live-donor nephrectomy	Robotic longer (sig)	Robotic shorter (sig)	0	NR	Similar	Horgan et al. 2002

Note: sig: significant; not sig: not significant; NR: not reported
Source: Reproduced by the author from Tooher and Pham (2004)

robotic surgery, and flag it as a low policy priority, in comparison to the application of laparoscopic surgery (Berkshire PCT 2007). It is obvious that economic evidence for the superiority of the robotic surgery needs to be explored urgently if it is to assume widespread adoption.

In essence, economic evaluation needs to define comparators; in our example, the comparators are open and conventional laparoscopic surgery. Cost and effectiveness should be calculated in an incremental way; and when clinical trial data is not available, or the long-term follow up is not applicable, economic models are required to simulate the situation and help in predicting the further development.

10.2. The Current State of Play of Economic Evaluation in Robotic Surgery

The three main features of economic evaluation studies on robotic surgery that have been carried out to date is that they are few in number, poor in quality, and biased in assessment endpoints.

10.2.1. Few Economic Studies in Robotic Surgery

There are few economic studies of surgery per se (Abrams and Wein 2000; Brazier and Johnson 2001), let alone in different surgical techniques, such as robotic surgery. A rapid search using the keyword "robot" in the National Health Service Economic Evaluation Database (NHS EED) produced 15 studies, of which only four can be classified as economic evaluation studies as shown in Table 10.3..

None of the above studies were conducted in the UK, and none of them were related to radical prostatectomy. The common features of these studies include:

TABLE 10.3. Economic evaluation studies of robotic surgery

Author	Year	Title	Country
Nakadi IE et al.	2006	Evaluation of da Vinci Nissen fundoplication, clinical results, and cost minimization	Belgium
Morino M et al.	2006	Randomized clinical trial of robotic-assisted versus laparoscopic Nissen fundoplication	Italy
Heemskerk J et al.	2005	First results after introduction of the four-armed da Vinci Surgical System in fully robotic laparoscopic cholecystectomy	Netherlands
Delaney CP et al.	2003	Comparison of robotically performed and traditional laparoscopic colorectal surgery	USA

- They were only cost-consequences studies and did not consider summarized effect measures such as quality of life;
- They were based on a small and insufficient sample size;
- They did not incorporate blind design;
- There was a lack of sample size calculation;
- And they did not include sensitivity analysis.

The quality of the above four studies is detailed in the next section.

A literature search in other databases with key terms such as "robot," "surgery," and "da Vinci™" generated several reviews (including protocols) and clinical trials of robotic surgery (Table 10.4.).

TABLE 10.4. Reviews and trials on robotic surgery

Database	Title	Author	Year	Type	Country
Cochrane Library	Robot assistant for laparoscopic **cholecystectomy**	Gurusamy KS et al.	2007	Review protocol	All
Ovid MEDLINE	Robotic-assisted versus conventional laparoscopic **fundoplication**: short-term outcome of a pilot randomized controlled trial	Muller-Stich BP et al.	2007	RCT	Germany
EMBASE	Laparoscopic radical **prostatectomy** for localized prostate cancer: A systematic review of comparative studies	Tooher R et al.	2006	Systematic review	Australia
Ovid MEDLINE	Evaluation of da Vinci **Nissen fundoplication** clinical results and cost minimization	Nakadi IE et al.	2006	RCT and economic evaluation	Belgium
Ovid MEDLINE	Randomized clinical trial of robotic-assisted versus laparoscopic Nissen **fundoplication**	Morino M et al.	2006	RCT	Italy

Ovid MEDLINE	**Gastrointestinal** robotic-assisted surgery. A current perspective	Lunca S et al.	2005	Review	Romania
Ovid MEDLINE	Robot-assisted *vs.* laparoscopic **adrenalectomy**: a prospective randomized controlled trial	Morino M et al.	2004	RCT	Italy
Ovid MEDLINE	Robotic-assisted **abdominal** surgery			Review	Germany
Ovid MEDLINE	What have we learnt after two years working with the da Vinci robot system in **digestive surgery**?			Review	Belgium

The common conclusion from these reviews and clinical trials was that there is no significant difference in the patients' health outcome. What is clearly needed is more definitive evidence for the benefits (or lack of them) of robotic surgery particularly through well-designed randomized controlled trials (RCT). One of the biggest problems in conducting a RCT is to recruit and randomize a sufficient number of patients to either the control group or the experimental group. This is discussed further in Section 10.2.4. Also, trial-based "piggyback" economic evaluation is needed together with a longer-term follow-up and a measure of patients' quality of life. Again, there is a lack of UK-based studies in these areas.

10.2.2. Poor Quality of Economic Studies

As mentioned above, to date, the quality of the current economic studies has been poor. Most studies are cost-consequences studies, which means there is no summary measure and comparison of cost and effectiveness. Instead, studies conducted to date have presented cost and results in itemized tables (Pizzi and Lofland 2006) as summarized in Table 10.5..

10.2.3. Fallacies in the Assessment of Robotic Surgery

- "Clinical Outcome ONLY" Fallacy

When one evaluates the efficacy of robotic surgery, one needs to first look at the reasons for the development of the robotic surgery. Robotic surgery was initially developed to solve the problem of reduced dexterity and impaired visual control: two inherited shortcomings of the conventional laparoscopic surgery. Therefore, one needs to measure if robotic surgery, in comparison with conventional open and laparoscopic techniques, has increased dexterity and

TABLE 10.5. Characteristics of the economic studies

Author	Year	Study Design	Control Group	Random-ization	Blinded design	Power calculation	Sample size	Sensitivity analysis	Postsurgery follow-up
Nakadi IE et al.	2006	Cost-consequences	Yes	Not sure	No	No	Small	No	12 months
Morino M et al.	2006	Cost-consequences	Yes	Yes	No	No	Small	No	12 months
Heemskerk J et al.	2005	Cost-consequences	Yes	No	No	No	Small	No	2 weeks
Delaney CP et al.	2003	Cost-consequences	No	No	No	Yes—But retrospectively	Small	No	No

improved visual control. By solving the problems of reduced dexterity and impaired visual control, the accuracy of the operation is "expected" to increase, the surgeon's learning curve reduced, and the fatigue of the surgeon lessened. In addition, more complicated procedures, that would not be ordinarily be performed by the conventional laparoscopic surgery, could be performed. The assessment should first address if these aims are achieved, through measuring outcomes that are directly related to these aims.

How does one measure increased dexterity and improved visual control? The technical teams who design these devices are best placed to achieve these aims, but only the surgeons who perform both procedures are able to tell the difference in practice. One direct measure of increased dexterity and visual control is to compare surgeons' learning and operation experiences. Ideally, the comparison should be performed among two groups of surgeons who have similar baseline characteristics, e.g., gender, age, education and training background, etc.

Take prostatectomy as an example: surgeons are to be divided into two groups. One group learns conventional laparoscopic prostatectomy, and another learns robotic-assisted prostatectomy. The aim is to detect differences in the surgeon's learning curves, fatigue and stress levels among surgeons, operation time, patients' blood loss, and length of hospital stay; patients' postsurgery potency and continence rate can also be linked to the accuracy in operation.

It is true that the ultimate goal of these technical advances is to improve patients' clinical outcomes, and to economize health resources, otherwise there is no justification of the increased cost of the robotic surgery. However, at the early stage of the assessment of new technologies, the measure of "clinical advantages" needs to focus on the outcomes that have the strongest causal link with the improved technical designs of robotic surgery.

Many clinical outcomes depend on factors other than the advancement of surgical techniques, for example, the post-surgery pain level, measured by the amount of analgesia used, is mainly influenced by surgeons' preferences. These factors will be overlooked if there are no RCTs to rule out potential bias in the assessment. Increased dexterity and visual control would presumably help surgeons to improve their ability in maneuvering during the operation, for example, by increasing the accuracy and the speed of incisions and sutures. In this way, the trauma caused by less accurate and less rapid conventional techniques would be minimized, which should contribute to a quicker recovery and fewer postoperative complications for patients.

In summary, at least four endpoints from the patients' perspective need to be highlighted: blood loss, operation time, length of hospital stay, and postoperative continence and potency rate.

The economic values of the above-mentioned endpoints include costing blood loss, operation time, length of hospital stay, and pre/postoperative patients' Quality Adjusted Life Years (QALY) (measured by, for example, EQ-5D). Furthermore, the improved surgeon's experience can be evaluated through measuring the surgeon's fatigue and stress levels.

- "Learning Curve for ALL" Fallacy

Among the few studies that examine the learning curve of robotic surgery, none has taken into account the previous experience and other characteristics of the surgeons under study. For example, for a surgeon who has performed open surgeries for many years, the learning curve of robotic surgery would be very different from that of a novice surgeon who has only performed a few open surgeries, and would also be different from a surgeon who is experienced in laparoscopic surgery.

As noted in the section of outcome measures below, it would be most appropriate to compare "surgeons alike," and to train surgeons from the beginning for this new technique. However, this would be difficult from a practical perspective as most surgeons have acquired certain skills before they take up robotic surgery. Therefore, it is important to recognize that combining surgeons of different "characteristics" will disguise the true learning and operating time required by the surgeons. Nevertheless, it is still likely that surgeons are grouped according to their varied past experience, and this may contribute to the knowledge of the association between surgeons' characteristics and the learning curve. Once this is explored, different specialized and focused training programmes could be designed and employed for different subgroups to achieve the optimal training effect. In summary, there is no single "learning curve" for all surgeons; and the learning curve is a parameter of the surgeons' characteristics. The economic implication of this "learning curve" measure is vital since the cost attached to the different training time and programmes could be substantial.

10.2.4. The Challenges of Economic Evaluation in Robotic Surgery

It was noted above that there are certain difficulties in collecting evidence in this area, a number of specific issues are now discussed. The conventional practice of economic evaluation of health interventions is to analyze "piggy-back" economic data directly obtained from well-conducted clinical trials. However, first of all, randomized controlled clinical trials are seldom carried out in this area, partly due to the difficulty of recruiting and randomizing patients up to a sufficient sample size to detect significant difference in health outcomes brought by different surgical techniques; secondly, long-term data on the cost and effectiveness of the new techniques is not available; and thirdly, there is a lack of consistency on the outcome measures, for example, the threshold measure for the positive margin could vary.

- Sample Size, the Recruitment and Randomization of Patients

Given the likely small or even insignificant differences in patients' clinical outcomes brought by robotic and conventional surgical techniques, the problem in relation to the sample size and study power calculation has been well recognized, as mentioned in Section 10.2.1. This is because one requires a relatively large sample to show the significant difference in certain clinical outcomes, for example, mortality rate.

- Long-Term Follow-Up Data

Since robotic surgery technology has been in place for only a few years, long-term follow-up data are not available. In addition, in the long run, with improvement in techniques, updated software and more ergonomic design, the impact on patients in the postoperative follow-up period is likely to change.

- Different Standards of Outcome Measure Thresholds

Different thresholds in outcome measures are prevalent in studies conducted to date, with the thresholds varying most significantly by the settings the study was conducted in. For example, the benign surgical positive margin, an important oncologic outcome, can be linked and sectioned according to different protocols which may lead to different positive margin results. Postsurgery continence can be defined as 0–1 pad (*safety pad*) or "No pad"; potency can be measured by sexual intercourse, return to baseline, or IIEF >21. The length of stay could also be biased if surgeons are keen to get patients out of the hospital to show the advantages of robotic surgery.

If these comparative thresholds are not standardized, the outcome measure could be seriously biased, rendering the economic evaluation invalid.

In summary, there are significant shortcomings in the economic evaluations of robotic surgery that have been conducted to date which reflect lack of good quality clinical and patient response data for the effect of the technology. Future economic evaluations in this area should rely more on economic modeling, which would help decision makers understand the trade-offs between alternative options different uncertainty levels.

Economic modeling of surgery techniques recognizes that it is easier to define and measure costs than to measure effectiveness. The cost items usually consist of the cost of the robotic device and associated facilities, operation staff time, etc. The effectiveness is usually measured by the health outcome attributable to the surgery, e.g., efficacy and safety results.

In the following section, relevant issues are clarified with the aim to address the challenges in economic evaluation. The radical prostatectomy is used as an example to demonstrate the different economic evaluation methods and to populate a decision model.

10.3. Further Suggestions and Decision Modeling in Economic Evaluation of Robotic Surgery

Acknowledging the shortcomings of economic evaluations of robotic surgery that have been performed to date, it is time to map the future development in this area, following a brief review of economic evaluation disciplines.

10.3.1. Evaluation Question and Subjects

The evaluation question, as noted in this chapter, is the comparison of costs and effectiveness of different surgical technologies: open, conventional laparoscopic, and robotic surgery. The effectiveness measure can include both patients' clinical endpoints and surgeons' experience outcomes. Ideally the evaluation subjects should embrace both patients and surgeons, but the preliminary model only considers the patients' outcome.

10.3.2. Assessment Measures

The assessment instruments and measures are used to quantify the clinical and economic endpoints. For example, the EQ-5D can be used to measure the effectiveness in terms of patients' experience and satisfaction; the International Index of Erectile Function (IIEF) is a measure of postsurgery potency. Standards need to be set for these measures.

10.3.3. Economic Evaluation Designs

Conventionally, there are four main types of economic evaluations: cost-minimization (CMA), cost-effectiveness (CEA), cost-utility (CUA), and cost-benefit analysis (CBA). Some text books add one more type: "cost-consequences" analysis (CCA). CMA can be viewed as a special type of CCA since both do not have a summarized comparison between costs and consequences, i.e., in CCA, costs and consequences are separately presented, if the consequences of interest are similar, then CMA is applied to compare the costs.

CEA is one of the most popular analytical methods used in clinical trials owing to its simplicity in the definition of costs and effectiveness. However, a limitation of CEA is also inherent in this simplicity in that it can only compare the same type of consequences, e.g., the blood pressure. When it comes to decision-making about interventions that bring about different types of clinical outcomes, a more comprehensive measure of endpoints, such as Quality Adjusted Life Years, is required. QALY is essentially a generic measure of a person's health utility, and can be compared among different interventions in CUA. A further step in health policy decision-making is to assign monetary value to the health and utility gain, this introduces an important decision threshold measure in CBA: the Net Monetary Benefit (NMB), using the combination of NMB and with Willingness to Pay (WTP), decision makers can easily choose between alternatives from an economic perspective and can also clearly justify the trade-offs.

Nevertheless, there are arguments about QALY as a measure of utility, and the rationale of attaching monetary values to utility (Kahneman 2005), although there are few alternatives available to replace such a measure at this time.

Another interesting discussion around the economic evaluation techniques centers on the use of Frequentist or Bayesian statistical analysis. Put simply, the major difference between these two techniques is that the Frequentist approach conducts analysis in a "laboratory" way, which puts unrealistic "context-free" assumptions at the baseline; whilst the Bayesian approach does not assume a "vacuum" environment, and tends to gather subjective probabilities in "real situations." The Bayesian approach is closely linked to the decision analytical modeling and expected utility theory (Spiegelhalter et al. 2003).

As for the current economic evaluation of robotic surgery, since it is highly unlikely to recruit and randomize patients into open surgery or robotic groups, "piggy-back" economic evaluation within a randomized clinical trial is not the ideal option (as discussed in section 10.2.4). In addition, trial-based economic evaluation has certain limitations, for example, the clinical data collection sometimes does not satisfy the economic data requirements, as noted by Claxton et al. (2002). Economic modeling therefore seems to offer an opportunity to gather systematically the most available information in multilevel simulation, by taking into account the uncertainty through advanced sensitivity analysis, and to eventually supply reliable predictions of the range of true values.

10.3.4. *Economic Modeling in Decision Making—Robotic-Assisted Radical Prostatectomy*

This section prepares a simple example of economic modeling and decision analysis of radical prostatectomy: open, laparoscopic, and robotic surgery. Since data of many clinical and economic endpoints is still insufficient to be statistically reliable (and is possibly inaccurate), a number of assumptions are made based on the information obtained from discussions with experts. These assumptions are clearly subject to challenge and debate from different information sources. Notwithstanding this, the economic model can help in building a preliminary structure of current economic evaluation, and may contribute to the framework in the development of economic evaluation of robotic surgery.

As stated by Drummond et al. (2005), the decision analytical modeling has five important objectives: (1) to supply a structure that reflects the treatment impact on the individual's prognoses, (2) to bring together relevant evidence, (3) to translate the evidence into estimates of the cost and effects of the alternative comparators, (4) to assess the various types of uncertainty in the evaluation, and (5) to identify future research priorities.

The model building process follows a suggested checklist for assessing quality in decision analytic models by Philips et al. (2004). The analysis is conducted in TreeAge ProSuite version 2007.

10.3.4.1. Decision Problem

The objective of the evaluation is to compare the cost-effectiveness of the three surgical techniques in prostatectomy: open, laparoscopic, and robotic-assisted.

10.3.4.2. Evaluation Perspective

The perspective of the model, i.e., the relevant costs and consequences, is the societal perspective since it is the most comprehensive perspective of health resource allocation. The societal perspective involves the cost and consequences related to the healthcare provider, patients, and society.

10.3.4.3. Model Structure

The model structure is shown in Fig. 10.1.

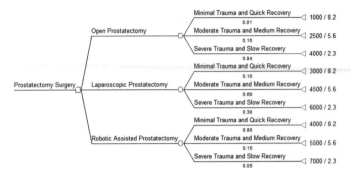
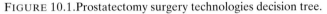

FIGURE 10.1. Prostatectomy surgery technologies decision tree.

10.3.4.4. Structure Assumptions

Considering the specific characteristics in relation to the prostatectomy surgery technology (see the discussion in Section 10.2), the clinical endpoints included in the effect branches are: blood loss, length of hospital stay (LOS), time before removal of catheter, time before return back to normal activity after removal of catheter, 3-month postsurgery continence rate, and 6-month postsurgery potency rate.

10.3.4.5. Comparators

The comparators are the robotic-assisted radical prostatectomy, the open radical prostatectomy, and the conventional laparoscopic radical prostatectomy.

10.3.4.6. Model Type

A simplified "decision tree" of the probabilistic cost-effectiveness model is constructed; the structure of the model is presented in 10.3.4.3. Ideally, in order to present the probability of postsurgery recurrence of cancer and long-term treatment effect and quality of life, a Markov model needs to be fitted in a more comprehensive decision tree. However, a Markov model is not constructed in this chapter since (1) the information about the long-term treatment effect of the surgical procedures is not yet available, and (2) the long-term difference in the recurrence rates under different surgical technologies is presumed not to be significantly different (Lepor 2006). Nevertheless, if and when such data becomes available, the Markov model could certainly be introduced into the economic model.

10.3.4.7. Time Frame

Consistent with the above justification of model type, the time horizon is limited to 12-months postsurgery. This implies that the duration of the treatment effect is followed up to one year, whilst the duration of the treatment is the average operation time, e.g., 200 minutes.

10.3.4.8. Disease Pathways

The "disease pathways" is a series of chance nodes that characterize the effects of the alternative strategies, as shown in the model structure (Fig. 10.1) through a series of branches representing particular events, which includes "Minimal Trauma and Quick Recovery," "Moderate Trauma and Medium Recovery," and "Severe Trauma and Slow Recovery."

The selection of the different clinical endpoints to be combined in three main effect pathways is consistent with the rationale in Section 10.2. Since there is limited literature on the threshold of clinical endpoints (Ficarra et al. 2007), the selection of the endpoint thresholds is rather arbitrary and is as follows:

- Minimal Trauma and Quick Recovery:

    Blood loss ≤ 150 ml
    Length of stay (LOS) ≤ 1 day
    Removal of catheter (RC) ≤ 3 days;
    Back to normal activity ≤ 5 days after RC;
    3-month postsurgery continence rate $\geq 90\%$
    6-month postsurgery potency rate $\geq 70\%$

- Moderate Trauma and Medium Recovery:

  150 ml < Blood loss ≤300 ml
  1 day < Length of stay ≤4 days
  3 days < Removal of catheter ≤6 days;
  5 days < Back to normal activity ≤7 days after RC;
  3-month post 70% ≤ surgery continence rate <90%
  50% ≤ 6-month postsurgery potency rate <70%

- Severe Trauma and Slow Recovery:

  300 ml < Blood loss ≤500 ml
  4 day < Length of stay ≤7 days
  6 days < Removal of catheter ≤9 days;
  7 days < Back to normal activity ≤10 days after RC;
  3-month post 40% ≤ surgery continence rate <70%
  30% ≤6-month postsurgery potency rate <50%

As shown in the model structure, probabilities of each clinical pathway for each surgical technology are set at:

- Open: Minimal Trauma and Quick Recovery—1%; Moderate Trauma and Medium Recovery—15%; Severe Trauma and Slow Recovery—84%.
- Laparoscopic: Minimal Trauma and Quick Recovery—10%; Moderate Trauma and Medium Recovery—60%; Severe Trauma and Slow Recovery—30%.
- Robotic: Minimal Trauma and Quick Recovery—80%; Moderate Trauma and Medium Recovery—15%; Severe Trauma and Slow Recovery—5%.

10.3.4.9. Data: Identification, Modeling, and Incorporation

Most data, at this stage, is derived from the current literature and expert opinions. The data source is rather limited. More validated data is required.

10.3.5. Costs

Item cost is not calculated; instead, the summary of cost for each clinical pathway is estimated, based on limited evidence (Mouraviev et al. 2007). Since the model is built with the society perspective, the cost integrates patients' cost and societal resource cost, as well as direct cost items relevant to the different surgical technology, such as purchase and maintenance of facilities, operation, hospital stay, medication, post-surgery services, etc. The summary of the cost, as presented in Fig. 10.1, is as follows:

- Open: Minimal Trauma and Quick Recovery—£1000; Moderate Trauma and Medium Recovery—£2500; Severe Trauma and Slow Recovery—£4000
- Laparoscopic: Minimal Trauma and Quick Recovery—£3000; Moderate Trauma and Medium Recovery—£4500; Severe Trauma and Slow Recovery—£6000
- Robotic: Minimal Trauma and Quick Recovery—£4000; Moderate Trauma and Medium Recovery—£5500; Severe Trauma and Slow Recovery—£7000

10.3.5.1. Effects and Quality of Life Measures

QALY is assumed to vary depending on different clinical pathways: for Minimal Trauma and Quick Recovery, QALY is 8.2; for Moderate Trauma and Medium Recovery, QALY is 5.6; for Severe Trauma and Slow Recovery, QALY is 2.3.

10.3.5.2. Uncertainty and Sensitivity Analysis

There are four major types of uncertainty in the analysis in relation to (1) analytical methods and steps (methodological), (2) model structure (structural), (3) sampling process and sample characteristics (heterogeneity), and (4) variables and data (parameter). In our hypothetical sample, we presume that the heterogeneity is not present as the baseline characteristics of the patients are assumed to be similar. The sensitivity analyses of methodological and structural uncertainty require alternative models, which are not available in the current scenario, but deserve further exploration through development of different models. Therefore, only the sensitivity analysis of parameter uncertainty is carried out by varying the Willingness to Pay value.

10.3.5.3. Internal and External Consistency

This is a process of checking the internal accuracy of mathematical logic and the external representativeness of the results in different settings. Both are beyond the scope of this section where only simple modeling structure is introduced. Nevertheless, the consistency assessment is a required component in formal economic modeling papers and the decision-making process.

10.3.5.4. Summary of the Results of Modeling

- Cost-Effectiveness Analysis (Table 10.6. and Fig. 10.2)

  ICER = IC/IE
  (ICER: Incremental Cost-Effectiveness Ratio; IC: Incremental Cost; IE: Incremental Effectiveness)
  Noted from Table 10.6 and Fig. 10.2. is that "laparoscopic prostatectomy" and "open prostatectomy" are dominated by "robotic prostatectomy." Therefore, robotic prostatectomy is the dominant strategy, i.e., more effective and less costly.

- Net Monetary Benefit and Willingness to Pay

  NMB = E*WTP—C
  (E: Effectiveness; C: cost)
  The WTP is set at £30 K; the NMB of different technologies is shown in Table 10.7. It appears that Robotic Prostatectomy has the highest NMB at the WTP = £30 K/QALY level.

TABLE 10.6. Cost and effectiveness of prostatectomy techniques

Strategy	Cost	IC	Effectiveness	IE	C/E	ICER
Open prostatectomy	£3745.0		2.85 QALYs		£1312/QALY	
Laparoscopic prostatectomy	£4800.0	£425.0	4.87 QALYs	−2.65 QALYs	£986/QALY	Dominated
Robotic-assisted prostatectomy	£4375.0	£630.0	7.51 QALYs	4.66 QALYs	£582/QALY	Dominate (£135/QALY)

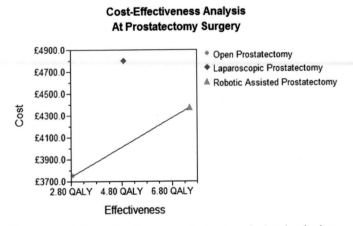

FIGURE 10.2. Cost-effectiveness analysis of surgical technologies.

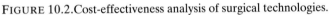

TABLE 10.7. NMB at WTP = 30 K/QALY

Strategy	NMB
Open	70 K
Laparoscopic	140 K
Robotic	220 K

- Simple sensitivity analysis with the different WTP thresholds.

Robotic prostatectomy has the highest NMB value at different WTP thresholds (Fig. 10.3.).

- Monte Carlo simulation for sensitivity analysis.

Monte Carlo simulation (Table 10.8.) is a popular method in Probabilistic Sensitivity Analysis (PSA). PSA is developed to overcome the drawbacks of simple sensitivity analysis (Drummond et al. 2005). In Monte Carlo simulation,

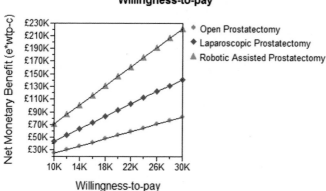

FIGURE 10.3.Sensitivity analysis of NMB at WTP thresholds: £10 K–£30 K/QALY.

many sets (e.g., 1000 sets in TreeAge) of expected costs and effects are run randomly to reflect the combined parameter uncertainty in the model. The following shows several results in the simulation.

The incremental cost-effectiveness (ICE) (Fig. 10.4.) of two strategies can be plotted in the ICE scatterplot. The sharp ellipse-shaped area shows the range of the incremental cost and effectiveness of two comparators: comparing to the laparoscopic prostatectomy, the interval of incremental cost of robotic prostatectomy is between –£2000 and £1000, whilst the incremental effectiveness is between 0 QALY and 6 QALY.

The relative concentration of the points in the scatterplot can be detected visually from the 3-D mountain graph (Fig. 10.5.). The concentration level supplies supplementary information of the ICE, the higher the concentration, the stronger the evidence.

The top vertical light-blue area denotes that the points in the ICE scatterplot are highly concentrated; this means the

TABLE 10.8. Monte Carlo simulation of cost, effectiveness, and NMB (random run: 1000; method: micro-simulation)

Statistic	Cost (Open)	Effect (Open)	NMB (Open)	Cost (Lapa)	Effect (Lapa)	NMB (Lapa)	Cost (Rob)	Effect (Rob)	NMB (Rob)
Mean	£3751	2.8 yrs	£81452	£4804	4.9 yrs	£141187	£4369	7.5 yrs	£221498
Std Dev	£601	1.3 yrs	£39245	£880	1.8 yrs	£55198	£787	1.5 yrs	£44985
Minimum	£1000	2.3 yrs	£65000	£3000	2.3 yrs	£63000	£4000	2.3 yrs	£62000
2.50%	£2500	2.3 yrs	£65000	£3000	2.3 yrs	£63000	£4000	2.3 yrs	£62000
10%	£2500	2.3 yrs	£65000	£4500	2.3 yrs	£63000	£4000	5.6 yrs	£162500
Median	£4000	2.3 yrs	£165500	£4500	5.6 yrs	£163500	£4000	8.2 yrs	£242000
90%	£4000	5.6 yrs	£165500	£6000	5.6 yrs	£163500	£5500	8.2 yrs	£242000
97.50%	£4000	5.6 yrs	£245000	£6000	8.2 yrs	£243000	£7000	8.2 yrs	£242000
Maximum	£4000	8.2 yrs	£245000	£6000	8.2 yrs	£243000	£7000	8.2 yrs	£242000
Sum (n*mean)	£3751000	2840.1 yrs	£81452000	£4804500	4866.4 yrs	£141187500	£4369000	7528.9 yrs	£221498000

ICE Scatterplot of
Robotic Assisted Prostatectomy vs. Laparoscopic Prostatectomy

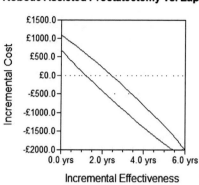

FIGURE 10.4.ICE scatterplot of robotic prostatectomy versus laparoscopic prostatectomy at WTP = £30 K.

Mountain Graph

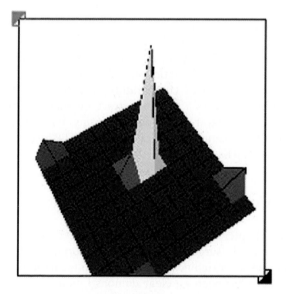

FIGURE 10.5.Mountain graph of ICE scatterplot at WTP = £30 K.

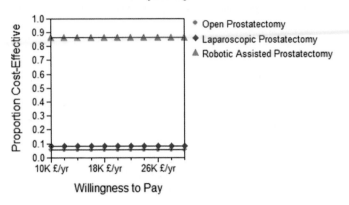

FIGURE 10.6. Cost-effectiveness acceptability curves.

dominance of robotic surgery over laparoscopic surgery is strongly supported.

- Acceptability curve.

The acceptability curve is a visual aid for decision analytical modeling. Information about the probability of Cost Effectiveness (CE) of comparators at different WTP levels can be viewed in a straightforward manner. Figure 10.6. demonstrates that robotic prostatectomy has the highest probability of being cost-effective at any WTP level between £10 K and £30 K.

10.4. Conclusions

In this chapter, the importance of the economic evaluation of robotic surgery is highlighted. Adoption of robotic surgery requires significant investment in technology and, to date, there has been no clear demonstration of its superior effectiveness relative to alternative techniques. Economic evaluation can be used to understand the link between cost and effectiveness and therefore can be useful in making evidence-based health policy decisions.

The current state-of-art in the economic evaluations of robotic surgery is reviewed in the second section. To date there have been very few economic studies, and most of them are low in quality. The efficacy studies are also subject to bias under uncontrolled trial design. The "insignificant" clinical results generated from these studies introduced further discussion of the "fallacies" in the assessment, and major obstacles in robust economic evaluation, namely, the problems associated with patient sample recruitment and randomization, the short follow-up period, and the nonstandardized thresholds in measuring some clinical endpoints.

Decision analytical modeling, currently, seems a more practical and promising method in answering the above challenges. In the third section, a probabilistic cost-effectiveness economic model is built using a simplified decision tree. The aim of building this model is not to detect the actual cost-effectiveness of the robotic surgery; instead, it serves as an example and supplies a framework of the process of model building, under the guidance of a standard protocol, based on which more comprehensive and advanced models can be constructed.

In this case, the clinical pathways and basic assumptions in the model are not strictly restricted to current knowledge; this also explains the unanimous results indicating the dominant cost-effectiveness of robotic surgery, compared to open and laparoscopic surgery. Caution has to be noted again: this model is a simulation of the model-building process, and is not ready to be used as a formal example of valid economic evaluation; hence the "simulated" results are highly unrealistic.

Further development of more advanced models should include the best-available evidence on clinical pathways and probabilities, the long-term health outcomes of patients, and the possibility and the rate of declining costs of the technology owing to economies of scale, etc.

The hypothetical decision modeling, populated with ideal-ized data, has an important predicative value through using the "roll-back" function. It can be used to help predict, if a certain level of economic dominance needs to be achieved, what the cost and effectiveness should be. While the eco-nomic evaluation of robotic surgery may be difficult at the time being it can be used to identify the sort of level of benefit that the technology will have to achieve if it is to be judged cost effective.

References

Anis AH, Gagnon Y (2000) Using economic evaluations to make formulary coverage decisions: so much for guidelines. Pharma-coEconomics 18:55–62

Abrams P, Wein A (2000) Recent advances: urology. BMJ 321: 1393–1396

Berkshire PCT Priority Committee (2007) Minutes of meet-ing held on Wednesday 4th July. Accessed on 15th April 2008 at: http://www.berkshire.nhs.uk/priorities/´policies/Minutes-4-July-2007.pdf

Brazier JE, Johnson AG (2001) Economics of surgery. The Lancet 358:1077–1081

Bucerius J, Metz S, Walther T, Falk V, Doll N, Noack F, Holzhey D, Diegeler A, Mohr F (2002) Endoscopic internal thoracic artery dissection leads to significant reduction of pain after minimally invasive direct coronary artery bypass graft surgery. Annals of Thoracic Surgery 73(4):1180–1184

Caceres F, Sanchez C, Martinez-Pineiro L, Tabernero A, Alonso S, Cisneros J, Cabrera Castillo PM, Alvarez Maestro M, Martin Hernandez M, Perez-Utrilla Perez M, de la Pena JJ (2007) Laparoscopic radical prostatectomy versus robotic. Archivos españoles de urología 60(4):430–438

Claxton K, Sculpher M, Drummond M (2002) A rational framework for decision making by the National Institute for Clinical Excel-lence. Lancet 360:711–715

Commonwealth of Australia (1995) Guidelines for the pharmaceu-tical industry on preparation of submissions to the Pharmaceutical Benefits Advisory Committee: including economic analyses. Department of Health and Community Services, Canberra

Delaney CP, Lynch AC, Senagore AJ, Fazio VW (2003) Comparison of robotically performed and traditional laparoscopic colorectal surgery. Dis Colon Rectum 46(12):1633–1639

Drummond M, O'Brien B, Stoddart G, Torrance G (1997) Methods for the Economic Evaluation of Healthcare Programmes. Oxford University Press, Oxford, quoting William A (1986)

Drummond MF, Sculpher MJ, Torrance GW, O'Brien BJ, Stoddart GL (2005) Methods for the Economic Evaluation of Healthcare Programmes. 3rd ed. Oxford University Press, Oxford

Ficarra V, Cavaleri S, Novara G, Aragona M, Artibani W (2007) Evidence from robot-assisted laparoscopic radical prostatectomy: a systematic review. Eur Urol 51:45–56

Food and Drug Administration (1997) Food and Drug Modernization Act of 1997, section 114. Accessed on 14th April 2008 at: http://www.fda.gov/cder/guidance/105-115.htm

Gettman M, Peschel R, Neururer R, Bartsch G (2002). A comparison of laparoscopic pyeloplasty performed with the daVinci robotic system versus standard laparoscopic techniques: initial clinical results. Eur Urol 42(5):453–457

Giulianotti P, Coratti A, Angelini M, Sbrana F, Cecconi S, Balestracci T, Caravaglios G (2003) Robotics in general surgery: personal experience in a large community hospital. Arch Surg 138(7):777–784

Gurusamy KS et al. (2007) Robot assistant for laparoscopic cholecystectomy. Cochrane Database of Systematic Reviews, Issue 4

Heemskerk J, Van Dam R, Van Gemert WG, Beets GL, Greve JW, Jacobs MJ, Bouvy ND (2005) First results after introduction of the four-armed da Vinci Surgical System in fully robotic laparoscopic cholecystectomy. Digest Surg 22(6):426–431

Horgan S, Vanuno D, Sileri P, Cicalese L, Benedetti E (2002) Robotic-assisted laparoscopic donor nephrectomy for kidney transplantation. Transplantation 73(9):1474–1479

Kahneman D (2005) Determinants of health economic decisions in actual practice: the role of behavioural economics. A summary of a presentation given by Prof. Daniel Kahneman at the ISPOR 10th Annual Int Meet First Plenary Session. Value in Health 9(2):65–67

Krahn M (1999) Principles of economic evaluation in surgery. World J Surg 23:1242–1248

Lepor H (2006) Open versus robotic radical prostatectomy. Urol Oncol Sem Orig Investig 24:91–93

Lotan Y, Cadeddu JA, Gettman MT (2004) The new economics of radical prostatectomy: cost comparison of open, laparoscopic and robot assisted techniques. The J Urol 172:1431–1435

Lunca S, Bouras G, Stanescu AC (2005) Gastrointestinal robot-assisted surgery. A current perspective. Romanian J Gastroenterol 14(4):385–391

McGuire A (2006) Theoretical concepts in the economic evaluation of healthcare. In: Drummond M, McGuire A (eds) Economic Evaluation in Healthcare: Merging Theory with Practice. Oxford University Press, Oxford

Melvin W, Needleman B, Krause K, Schneider F, Ellison E (2002) Computer-enhanced vs standard laparoscopic antireflux surgery. J Gastroint Surg 6(1):11–16

Menon M, Tewari A, Baize B, Guillonneau B, Vallancien G (2002) Prospective comparison of radical retropubic prostatectomy and robot-assisted anatomic prostatectomy: the Vattikuti Urology Institute experience. Urology 60(5):864–868

Morino M, Beninca G, Giraudo G, Del Genio GM, Rebecchi F, Garrone C (2004) Robot-assisted vs laparoscopic adrenalectomy: a prospective randomized controlled trial. Surg Endoscopy 18(12):1742–1746

Morino M, Pellegrino L, Giaccone C, Garrone C, Rebecchi F (2006) Randomized clinical trial of robot-assisted versus laparoscopic Nissen fundoplication. Brit J Surg 93(5):553–558

Mouraviev V, Nosnik I, Sun L, Robertson CN, Walther P, Albala D, Moul JW, Polascik TJ (2007) Financial comparative analysis of minimally invasive surgery to open surgery for localized prostate cancer: a single-institution experience. Urology 69(2): 311–314

Muhlmann G, Klaus A, Kirchmayr W, Wykypiel H, Unger A, Holler E, Nehoda H, Aigner F, Weiss HG (2003) DaVinci robotic-assisted laparoscopic bariatric surgery: Is it justified in a routine setting? Obesity Surg 13(6):848–854

Muller-Stich BP, Reitr MA, Wente MN, Bintintan VV, Koninger J, Buchler MW, Gutt CN (2007) Robot-assisted versus conventional laparoscopic fundoplication: short term outcome of a pilot randomized controlled trial. Surg Endosc 21(10):1800–1805

Nakadi IE, Melot C, Closset J, DeMoor V, Betroune K, Feron P, Lingier P, Gelin M (2006) Evaluation of da Vinci Nissen fundoplication clinical results and cost minimization. World J Surg 30(6):1050–1054

National Institute for Clinical Excellence (2004) Guide to the Methods of Technology Appraisal. NICE, London

Philips Z, Ginnelly L, Sculpher M et al. (2004) A review of guidelines for good practice in decision-analytic modeling in health technology assessment. Health Technol Assess 8(36):1–158

Pizzi L, Lofland JH (2006) Economic Evaluation in U.S. Healthcare: Principles and Applications. Jones and Bartlett Publishers, Sudbury, Massachusetts, p. 16

Spiegelhalter DJ, Abrams KR, Myles JP (2003) Bayesian Approaches to Clinical Trials and Health-care Evaluation. Wiley, Chichester

Tewari A, El-Hakim A, Leung RA (2006) Expert Rev Anticancer Ther 6(1):11–20

Tooher R, Pham C (2004) Technology Overview: da Vinci Surgical Robotic System. July 2004. Australian Safety and Efficacy Register of New Interventional Procedures—Surgical (ASERNIP-S). Accessed on 1st Nov 2007 at: http://www. surgeons.org/AM/Template.cfm?Section=Search˙Asernips&section =Technogy˙overviews&template=/CM/ContentDisplay.cfm& ContentFileID=7771

Tooher R, Swindle P, Woo H, Miller J, Maddern G (2006) Laparoscopic radical prostatectomy for localized prostate cancer: A systematic review of comparative studies. J Urol 175(6):2011–2017

TreeAge Prosuite (2007) TreeAge Software Inc. Accessed on 14th April 2008 at: http://www.treeage.com/products/overviewSuite. html

WHO (1998) Terminology—A glossary of technical terms on the economics and finance of health services. Regional Office for Europe, 1998 (document EUR/ICP/CARE0401/CN01)

Index

Note: The letter '*t*' *and* '*f*' in the index locators refer to tables and figures respectively.

Printed in the United States of America